Lipid disorders

YOUR QUESTIONS ANSWERED

John Reckless
DSc MD FRCP
Consultant Physician and Endocrinologist
Royal United Hospital, Bath
Honorary Reader in Medicine,
University of Bath, Bath, UK

Jonathan Morrell
MA MB BChir FRCGP DCH DRCOG
General Practitioner and Hospital
Practitioner in Cardiology,
Hastings, UK

D1421636

ELSEVIER
CHURCHILL
LIVINGSTONE

EDINBURGH LONDON NEW YORK OXFORD PHILADELPHIA ST LOUIS SYDNEY TORONTO 2005

ELSEVIER
CHURCHILL
LIVINGSTONE

First published 2005

ISBN 0 4430 7481 X

British Library Cataloguing in Publication Data
A catalogue record for this book is available from the British Library

Library of Congress Cataloging in Publication Data
A catalog record for this book is available from the Library of Congress

Note
Knowledge and best practice in this field are constantly changing. As new research and experience broaden our knowledge, changes in practice, treatment and drug therapy may become necessary or appropriate. Readers are advised to check the most current information provided (i) on procedures featured or (ii) by the manufacturer of each product to be administered, to verify the recommended dose or formula, the method and duration of administration, and contraindications. It is the responsibility of the practitioner, relying on their own experience and knowledge of the patient, to make diagnoses, to determine dosages and the best treatment for each individual patient, and to take all appropriate safety precautions. To the fullest extent of the law, neither the publisher nor the authors assume any liability for any injury and/or damage to persons or property arising out of or related to any use of the material contained in this book.

The Publisher

Printed in China

Lipid disorders

YC

Cover image: Surface maps of the electrostatic potential around a cholesterol molecule. Cholesterol plays a crucial role in the synthesis of bile salts and hormones, and in transporting fats in the bloodstream. High blood levels of cholesterol are thought to raise the risk of atherosclerosis, the build-up of fatty deposits on artery walls and a major cause of heart attack and stroke.

Alfred Pasieka/SPL

For Elsevier

Commissioning Editor: Fiona Conn
Project Development Manager: Isobel Black
Project Manager: Nancy Arnott
Design Direction: George Ajayi
Illustration Manager: Bruce Hogarth
Illustrator: Chartwell

Lipid disorders

YC

Cover image: Surface maps of the electrostatic potential around a cholesterol molecule. Cholesterol plays a crucial role in the synthesis of bile salts and hormones, and in transporting fats in the bloodstream. High blood levels of cholesterol are thought to raise the risk of atherosclerosis, the build-up of fatty deposits on artery walls and a major cause of heart attack and stroke.

Alfred Pasieka/SPL

For Elsevier

Commissioning Editor: Fiona Conn
Project Development Manager: Isobel Black
Project Manager: Nancy Arnott
Design Direction: George Ajayi
Illustration Manager: Bruce Hogarth
Illustrator: Chartwell

Contents

	Preface	vii
	How to use this book	ix
1	Lipid metabolism – the basics	1
2	Atherosclerosis, lipids and cardiovascular disease	17
3	Measuring lipids	37
4	Lipid disorders	47
5	Identifying individuals for treatment	65
6	Treatment by diet and lifestyle	77
7	Drug treatments for dyslipidaemia	99
8	Drug treatment – clinical trial evidence	129
9	Implementing best practice	139
10	Special situations	155
11	Economic aspects	167
12	New horizons – the next 10 years	173
	Appendix: Useful organisations and websites	181
	References	187
	Glossary of acronyms and abbreviations	197
	List of patient questions	199
	Index	201

Preface

The study of blood fats, or blood 'lipids', dates from the eighteenth century when cholesterol was first crystallised from alcoholic extracts of gall stones. Little did those early investigators realise that they had hit upon the central cause of arterial atherosclerosis, the disease process largely responsible for the modern epidemic of heart attacks and strokes. Most of us have heard of cholesterol but few realise how common it is to find abnormal blood levels. In truth, living in modern society, the majority of us have abnormal cholesterol levels and are potentially at risk from atherosclerotic disease. Sometimes raised levels are obvious, but in other situations the pattern of other blood lipids defines the risk and sometimes even apparently innocent levels benefit from modification.

In just a few decades, health professionals have witnessed the emergence of the study of blood lipids from theoretical science to the forefront of everyday clinical practice. A number of clinical trials have demonstrated that lipid lowering saves lives and prevents heart attacks and strokes, and health professionals are charged with implementing their findings. For a number of reasons, the implementation of the evidence base has been slow but a series of initiatives including new guidelines and directives, involving new structures and pathways of healthcare, have been set in place to redress this.

Inevitably, within an emerging and evolving discipline, a number of questions arise from interested health professionals and the public. At both personal and professional levels, this book aims, by answering a series of questions, to equip the reader with a comprehensive working knowledge of the subject. We hope, therefore, that the book will be useful to the range of health professionals who treat lipid disorders as well as the growing number of people who seek accurate, authoritative and unbiased information on which to base their personal health choices.

JR & JM

How to use this book

The *Your Questions Answered* series aims to meet the information needs of GPs and other primary care professionals who care for patients with chronic conditions. It is designed to help them work with patients and their families, providing effective, evidence-based care and management.

The books are in an accessible question and answer format, with detailed contents lists at the beginning of every chapter and a complete index to help find specific information.

ICONS
Icons are used in the book to identify particular types of information:

 highlights information important to clinical practice

 highlights side-effect information.

PATIENT QUESTIONS
At the end of relevant chapters there are sections of frequently asked patient questions, with easy-to-understand answers aimed at the non-medical reader. These questions are also listed at the end of the book.

Lipid metabolism – the basics

1

1.1	What is cholesterol?	2
1.2	What does cholesterol do?	2
1.3	What are triglycerides?	2
1.4	What do triglycerides do?	4
1.5	What are fatty acids and phospholipids?	4
1.6	What are lipoproteins?	5
1.7	How are lipoproteins classified?	6
1.8	What are apolipoproteins?	6
1.9	How is cholesterol synthesised?	8
1.10	How are cholesterol and triglycerides absorbed?	9
1.11	How are lipoproteins metabolised?	10
1.12	What role does LDL-cholesterol have in promoting atherosclerosis?	11
1.13	How does HDL-cholesterol protect against atherosclerosis?	11
1.14	Are triglycerides atherogenic?	12
1.15	What is the atherogenic lipoprotein phenotype?	13
1.16	What is lipoprotein(a)?	13

PQ PATIENT QUESTIONS

1.17	What are lipids?	14
1.18	Why is cholesterol important?	14
1.19	Where does cholesterol come from?	15
1.20	How much cholesterol do we need?	15
1.21	What is 'good' cholesterol?	15
1.22	What is 'bad' cholesterol?	15

1.1 What is cholesterol?

Cholesterol (*Fig. 1.1*) is a fat, a steroid molecule, which is largely insoluble in water. Some cholesterol is of dietary origin, but some cholesterol-derived sterols are also lost in the faeces. All cells are able to synthesise cholesterol, but nearly all cholesterol is synthesised in, and secreted from, the liver. Being a fat, cholesterol is then carried in blood in lipoproteins (*see Q 1.6*) to be available to peripheral tissues.

1.2 What does cholesterol do?

Cholesterol is an essential component of every cell's external membrane and of those of intracellular organelles, without which cells would not exist. The balance of free and esterified cholesterol, phospholipid (*see Q 1.5*), glycerides and membrane proteins ensures membrane integrity and stabilises membrane fluidity.

Cholesterol is also the precursor in the synthesis of steroid hormones, some fat-soluble vitamins and bile acids (*see Q 7.27*).

1.3 What are triglycerides?

Triglycerides (*Fig. 1.2*) are fats formed from fatty acids (*see Q 1.5*) and glycerol. Glycerol is formed from glucose. Glycerol has three carboxyl (COOH) groups on which one, two or three fatty acids are added (condensed) to give mono-, di- and triglycerides. Because there are many different fatty acids of different chain length and with different numbers of double bonds there are therefore many variations of triglycerides, and hence the usual use of the plural word. In the blood, fatty acids are also carried bound to albumin (i.e. not as triglycerides) and are then referred to as 'free fatty acids' or, more accurately, as 'non-esterified fatty acids'.

Dietary triglycerides are a substantial source for the total triglycerides in the body, but much body triglyceride is synthesised endogenously (within the body). Any superfluous components from body metabolism are recycled within the liver, and these metabolites are largely re-secreted into the blood as triglyceride or glucose and are then available for energy supply for tissues or for storage. Thus, a diet that may be low in fat (triglyceride) may contain calories superfluous for immediate need. Whether as simple sugars, complex carbohydrate, fat, protein or alcohol, these calorie sources will be substantially converted to triglyceride.

Stored triglyceride in adipose tissue is a very efficient fuel store. Adipose tissue is around 90% fat and at 9 calories per gram, 1 kg of

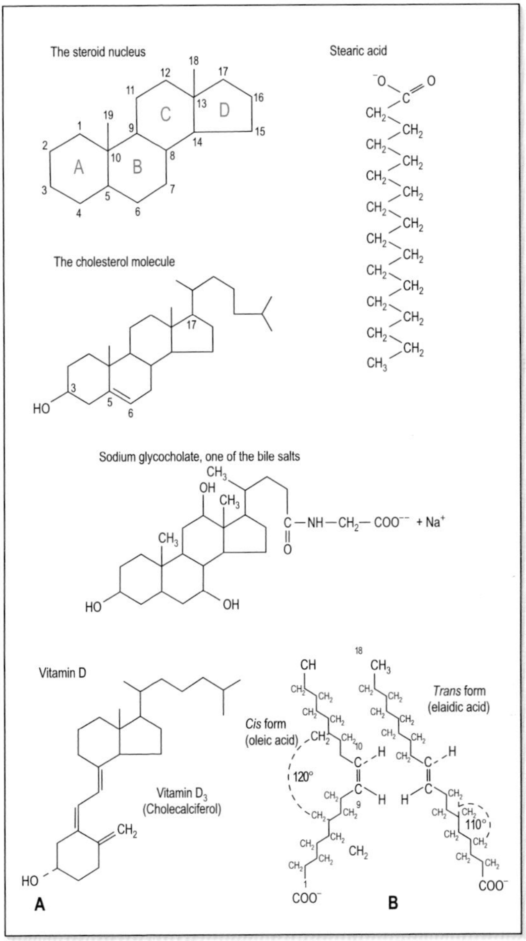

Fig. 1.1 Structures of fatty acids, cholesterol and related sterols. **A** From cholesterol, with various modest alterations to the basic steroid nucleus, are formed the sex hormones, bile acids and vitamin D. **B** Eighteen carbon fatty acids without a double bond (stearic acid) and with a single double bond (oleic acid). Where there are single bonds between carbon atoms rotation can occur and there is flexibility of fatty acid shape. At a double bond, however, there is a rigidity in the molecule introduced at this point. Depending on the configuration of the double bond introduced, one can have two shapes called *cis* and *trans* fatty acids (oleic acid and elaidic acid, respectively). In nature, almost all fatty acids are in the *cis* shape, excess *trans* fatty acids perhaps being harmful. *Trans* fatty acids can occur with hydrogenation of fats as may take place in the manufacture of some fat spreads, and can occur with recurrent heating of some cooking oils.

adipose tissues stores around 8000 calories. This contrasts with lean tissues with 80% water, where the glycogen or muscle protein yields around 4 calories per gram, 1 kg of lean tissue storing approximately 800 calories.

While glycerol is water soluble, fatty acids are substantially insoluble in water, particularly as chain length (the size of the fatty acid molecule) increases. Triglycerides are therefore largely water insoluble and, like cholesterol, are carried in the blood solubilised in much larger complex molecules – lipoproteins (*see* Q 1.5).

1.4 What do triglycerides do?

The primary role of triglycerides is as an energy source for body tissues, whether being dietary derived or endogenously (hepatically) synthesised.

From the gut, triglycerides are carried on chylomicrons (*see* Q 1.7), to peripheral tissues where the triglyceride may be hydrolysed, with the released fatty acids (*see* Q 1.5) being taken up for energy supply or for storage. The chylomicron remnant (*see* Q 1.7) is removed by the liver.

Triglycerides are synthesised in the liver from other available metabolites, and are secreted into the blood in very low density lipoproteins (VLDLs) (*see* Q 1.7), again for energy supply or storage, with the VLDL remnants (*see* Q 1.7) being converted to low density lipoproteins (LDLs) or returning to the liver.

Triglycerides also have roles in the structural integrity of cells.

1.5 What are fatty acids and phospholipids?

Fatty acids are chains of carbon atoms with hydrogen atoms on the side chains, and with a terminal carboxyl (COOH) group (*see Figs 1.1 and 1.2*). Fatty acids vary in the number of carbon atoms and in chain length; the longer the length the more insoluble they are in water. There may a double bond between two carbon atoms, each carbon losing a hydrogen atom – these are called 'unsaturated'. Fatty acids may be mono-unsaturated or poly-unsaturated depending on the number of double bonds (*see* Q 6.11).

Three fatty acids are condensed onto a glycerol 'backbone' to form triglycerides, which are the main 'fuel' storage for the body. The greater the number of unsaturated bonds the less solid the triglyceride is at room temperature. In adipose tissue the glycerol utilised is obtained from the metabolism of glucose.

Instead of one of the fatty acids, one of the three positions on the glycerol may be phosphorylated together with a compound such as choline or inositol to form a phospholipid. These are also important in cell function and in cell membrane structure.

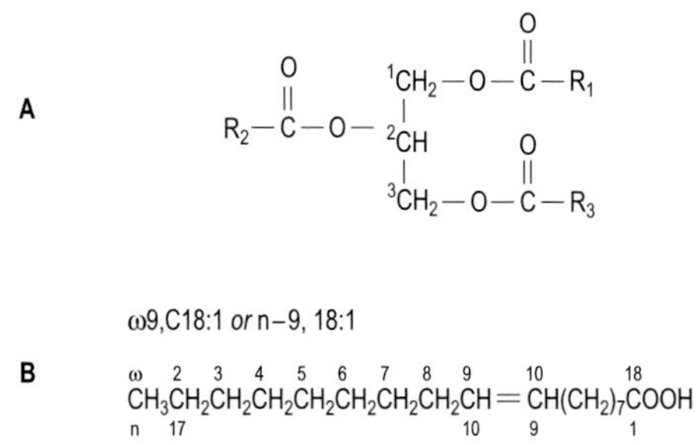

A

$$R_2-\overset{\overset{\displaystyle O}{\|}}{C}-O-\begin{array}{l}{}^{1}CH_2-O-\overset{\overset{\displaystyle O}{\|}}{C}-R_1 \\ {}^{2}CH \\ {}^{3}CH_2-O-\overset{\overset{\displaystyle O}{\|}}{C}-R_3\end{array}$$

$\omega 9, C18:1\ or\ n-9,\ 18:1$

B

$$\underset{n\ \ \ 17}{\overset{\omega\ \ 2\ \ \ 3\ \ \ \ 4\ \ \ 5\ \ \ 6\ \ \ 7\ \ \ 8\ \ \ 9}{CH_3CH_2CH_2CH_2CH_2CH_2CH_2CH_2CH}}=\underset{9\ \ \ \ \ \ \ \ \ \ \ \ 1}{\overset{10\ \ \ \ \ \ \ \ \ \ \ 18}{CH(CH_2)_7COOH}}$$

Fig. 1.2 Structure of triglyceride and fatty acids. **A** On the backbone of glycerol three fatty acids (R$_1$, R$_2$, R$_3$) are added to form a triglyceride molecule. The fatty acids vary in the number of carbon atoms they contain, being increasingly insoluble in water as the chain length increases. The number of double bonds between carbon atoms in the chain can also vary, from none (a saturated fatty acid) to one (monounsaturated) or two or more (polyunsaturated) (*see Fig. 1.1*). **B** The chemical structure of a typical fatty acid, oleic acid, is shown with one double bond. It is the carboxyl end of the molecule (–COOH) that attaches to glycerol in the formation of triglyceride. Different terminologies can be used to describe the structure. Here, the fatty acid has 18 carbons, and one double bond which is 9 carbon atoms away from the omega (ω) or n terminal end of the fatty acid. (CH$_2$)$_7$ is shorthand for seven repeats of CH$_2$.

In the blood, the 'free' fatty acids are carried largely bound to albumin as non-esterified fatty acids.

1.6   What are lipoproteins?

Lipoproteins are large, complex molecules designed to carry fats around the body in the blood. They are composed of various fats – cholesterol, cholesterol ester, phospholipid and triglyceride – and proteins which have both structural and functional roles. Most of the fat (cholesterol ester and triglyceride), being largely insoluble in water, is held in the core of the lipoprotein. Phospholipid and cholesterol have hydrophobic and hydrophilic domains and are orientated around the outer layer of the molecule with the water-favouring hydrophilic domain exposed on the lipoprotein surface. This allows the lipoprotein to be solubilised in the blood.

Different proteins are involved. Apolipoprotein-A (apo-A) is the main protein of high density lipoprotein (HDL), but the key structural molecule of all other lipoproteins is apolipoprotein-B (apo-B). Other important apolipoproteins are apo-C and apo-E (*see Q 1.8*).

1.7 How are lipoproteins classified?

Lipoproteins have been classified on the basis of their physical and chemical properties, and there are different methods for doing this.

> It is important to appreciate that a particular lipoprotein class does not consist of many identical molecules, but a whole range of sizes within that class (*Fig. 1.3*). Lipoproteins are synthesised not only in different numbers but also at different sizes depending on the amount of substrate (fats) to be moved around the body. As a lipoprotein circulates it changes size as components are lost or gained. Also, the relative percentage of individual components of the lipoprotein changes at the same time.

Ultracentrifugation separates lipoproteins on the basis of their relative density, with triglyceride-rich lipoproteins being lighter than cholesterol-rich lipoproteins. By far the largest and the lightest lipoproteins are the chylomicrons that are synthesised in the gut, and carry dietary fat from the gut to the peripheral tissues. The next largest particles are the VLDLs that carry liver-synthesised triglyceride and cholesterol to the peripheral tissues. VLDLs are converted to LDLs that provide cholesterol to cells. The remnant particles of chylomicrons and VLDLs are considered in 'lipoprotein metabolism' (*see* Q 1.11). Finally there are the HDLs, which are the smallest, densest particles.

Lipoproteins used to be classified by electrophoresis into alpha (HDL), beta (LDL) and pre-beta (VLDL) classes, related to their electrical charge and how far they moved on the electrophoresis gel. Large chylomicrons do not move and stay at the origin of the gel. This system has been largely abandoned for clinical care. Newer methods of separating and measuring individual lipoproteins have been and continue to be developed.

1.8 What are apolipoproteins?

Apo(lipo)proteins are the protein components of lipoproteins. They have both structural and functional roles.

- Apolipoprotein-A (two forms: apo-AI, apo-AII) is the main structural protein for HDL, and several molecules are present on each HDL particle.
- Apolipoprotein-B (apo-B) is the main structural protein for all the other lipoproteins, and there is just a single apo-B per lipoprotein that stays with the particle throughout its life.

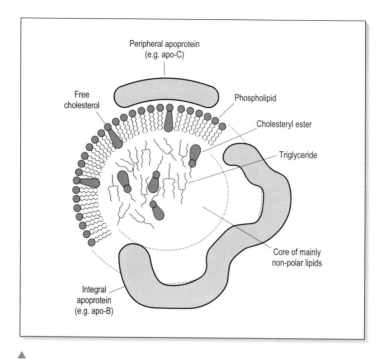

Fig. 1.3 The structure of a typical lipoprotein. Lipoproteins are complex molecules. The hydrophobic fat molecules, cholesterol ester and triglyceride, are in the core of the molecule. In addition to their major hydrophobic component, some fat molecules have a more hydrophilic portion, such as free cholesterol and phospholipids. These molecules are arranged around the outer surface of the lipoprotein, with the lipid component on the inside and the more water-soluble portion on the outside, which allows the whole lipoprotein to be soluble in a water environment in blood. There are a number of different protein components in lipoproteins which have both structural and functional roles. Apoprotein A is the structural protein for high density lipoprotein. Apoprotein B (apo-B) is the structural protein for all the other lipoproteins, also having a functional role for lipoprotein metabolism for all the apo-B containing lipoproteins except chylomicrons. apo-C, apoprotein C.

■ For liver-synthesised particles, a full length apo-B (apo-B100) also has a functional role, being required for the ultimate uptake of LDL into cells.

■ A truncated (48% of the whole molecule) version of apo-B (apo-B48) is on chylomicrons where there is a post-translational modification leading to the structural half of the protein only being made. As a result the chylomicron remnant follows a separate removal pathway in the liver, and does not bind to the apo-B receptor that recognises LDL.

■ Apo-C and apo-E move between lipoproteins and have functional roles. There are different apo-C subtypes that influence the fate of triglyceride-rich particles. Apo-CII is essential for the catabolism of the triglyceride-rich lipoproteins VLDL and chylomicrons. Apo-CII activates the enzyme lipoprotein lipase (LPL) that hydrolyses the triglyceride of triglyceride-rich lipoproteins. It also is needed for binding the lipoprotein to the activated LPL.

■ Apo-E allows recognition of triglyceride-rich lipoproteins and their remnants by hepatocytes, and therefore facilitates their removal.

1.9 How is cholesterol synthesised?

While some cholesterol is of dietary origin, and while all human cells are capable of making it, cholesterol is largely synthesised in the liver (*see Fig. 1.1*). From simple two carbon fragments are condensed longer molecules, 3-hydroxy-3-methylglutaryl-coenzyme-A (HMG-CoA) reductase being the last pluripotential step. HMG-CoA can be metabolised to other pathways, but activity of the enzyme HMG-CoA reductase leads to the formation of mevalonate. Multiple steps follow through isopentyl compounds (geranyl, farnesyl and geranylgeranyl groups) to squalene and ultimately through nearly 30 steps to the steroid nucleus and cholesterol (*Figs 1.4–1.6*). Other compounds of significance are derived from this pathway.

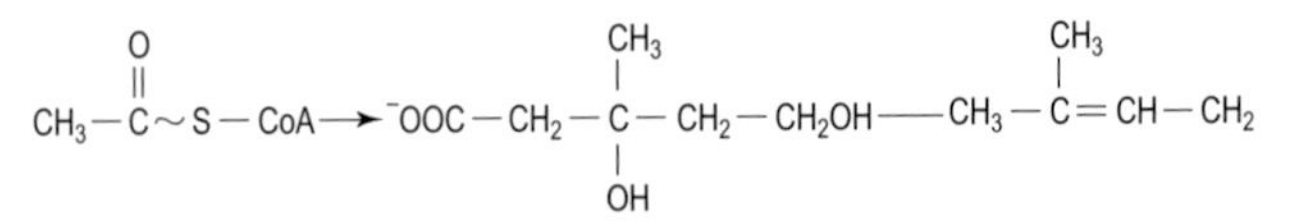

▲

Fig. 1.4 The synthetic pathway from short carbon chain molecules (acetoacetate) to cholesterol and related molecules. Acetyl-CoA is metabolised through a series of steps firstly to mevalonate, and then to 5-carbon isoprenoid units. It is at 3-hydroxy-3-methyl-glutaryl coenzyme-A (HMG-CoA), the step immediately prior to mevalonate, that the key drugs in treating high cholesterol work. These are the statins, inhibitors of the enzyme HMG-CoA reductase.

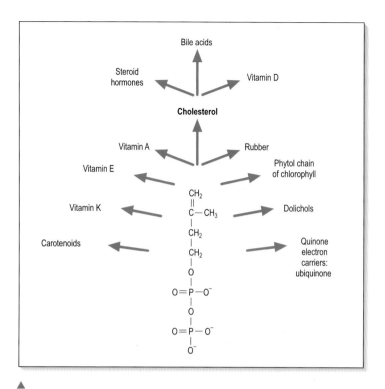

Fig. 1.5 The synthetic pathway from short chain carbon molecules to cholesterols and related molecules. The isoprenoid units (*see Fig. 1.4*) are phosphorylated and then condensed to form larger molecules prior to cholesterol; other key compounds are formed in both the plant and animal world.

1.10 How are cholesterol and triglycerides absorbed?

Dietary fats (triglycerides) are digested within the gut. In an alkaline environment they are hydrolysed by gut and pancreatic lipases to diglycerides, monoglycerides and free fatty acids, and with bile salts are emulsified and absorbed into the enterocyte as micelles. In the enterocyte, triglycerides are re-synthesised and with free and esterified cholesterol, phospholipid and a specific apolipoprotein (apo-B48; *see Q 1.8*) are secreted as chylomicrons (*see Q 1.7*) into the lymphatic system and then into the venous blood.

Cholesterol has a specific uptake mechanism, being taken across the enterocyte by a binding cassette protein. A recently introduced lipid-

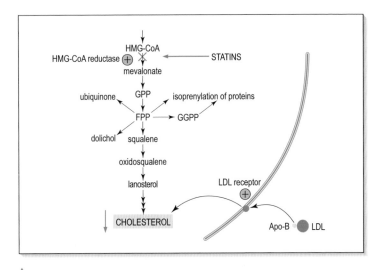

Fig. 1.6 Cholesterol is a complex molecule, but is synthesised from simple two- and four-carbon molecules through a pathway with multiple steps, a few of which are shown in the figure. Statins work by competitively blocking the key rate-limiting step in cholesterol synthesis, 3-hydroxy-3-methyl-glutaryl coenzyme-A (HMG-CoA) reductase. Until after the formation of mevalonic acid the products are pluripotential, so that limiting synthesis at the HMG-CoA reductase step will reduce subsequent flux through the pathway to cholesterol, but the HMG-CoA compound is utilised elsewhere. FPP, farensyl pyrophosphate; GGPP, geranylgeranyl pyrophosphate; GPP, geranyl pyrophosphate.

lowering drug (ezetimibe; *see Qs 7.21–7.23*) that partly blocks this transport pathway has increased our understanding of this process.

1.11 How are lipoproteins metabolised?

The triglycerides of chylomicrons are hydrolysed in peripheral tissues by the action of LPL. The glycerol component recycles to the liver, the fatty acids being taken up into tissues either for catabolism for energy supply or for re-synthesis into tissue triglyceride for energy storage. LPL, an insulin-sensitive enzyme, is synthesised in adipose tissue and muscle. It is activated by an apolipoprotein (apo-CII) carried on chylomicrons. The chylomicron shrinks in size and the liver removes the remnant.

The other triglyceride-rich lipoproteins are the VLDLs which carry triglyceride (and cholesterol) synthesised in the liver to peripheral tissues, where again LPL hydrolyses the triglyceride. The VLDL remnants are either removed by the liver as an intermediate density lipoprotein (IDL) or are converted to the main cholesterol carrying particles – LDLs.

LDLs – either directly synthesised by the liver or derived from VLDLs – deliver cholesterol to peripheral tissues where LDL is taken up by specific LDL receptors. Cells up- or down-regulate these receptors depending on their cholesterol need. Residual LDL (and usually half or more) is recycled to be removed by hepatic LDL receptors. These again are up- or down-regulated depending on cholesterol availability and need within the liver.

HDLs are synthesised as apo-A and phospholipid discs (nascent HDL) in liver (or gut) and on entry to the plasma take up cholesterol, cholesterol ester and other apolipoproteins to form mature HDL particles. In the circulation, HDL particles are able to stimulate cholesterol efflux from cholesterol-replete cells. Through the HDL-associated enzyme lecithin cholesterol acyl transferase (LCAT), this cholesterol is esterified, to be carried in the HDL core. HDL particles are able to offload cholesterol (as cholesterol ester) either onto circulating VLDL and LDL molecules or to hepatocytes. HDL particles repeat this process many times before being removed by liver or kidneys, apo-A being lost in the urine.

1.12 What role does LDL-cholesterol have in promoting atherosclerosis?

LDLs are required as a provider of cholesterol to body tissues, but only at low circulating amounts. Levels of <1 mmol/L that are present in the infant, rise in childhood and adulthood in all populations, but to a much greater level in westernised populations. In those areas of the world where populations have very low LDL-cholesterol levels, such as Japan and China,[1] the incidence of atherosclerotic clinical events is very low. These events rise steadily and markedly as circulating LDL levels rise in populations. One almost needs a certain amount of LDL cholesterol for atherogenesis, and without this even with other risk factors present atheroma is limited.

Excess circulating LDL causes endothelial abnormalities. LDL enters the arterial subintimal space where it is altered and oxidised, and where it is taken up by macrophages that then become the foam cell of the fatty streak and more advanced arterial lesions. The oxidised LDL and the activation of macrophages produce cytokines, and cell adhesion molecules are activated leading to further entry of monocytes between the endothelial cells into the subintimal space.

1.13 How does HDL-cholesterol protect against atherosclerosis?

HDL acts as a reverse cholesterol transport mechanism. HDL can accept cholesterol from cholesterol-replete cells, and return this cholesterol either to other lipoproteins (VLDLs and LDLs) in the circulation or to the liver for recycling.

HDL particles activate cell receptors, leading to hydrolysis of cholesterol ester and the mobilisation of the free cholesterol to the cell surface and onto the HDL. Here, the HDL-associated enzyme LCAT esterifies the cholesterol and the ester is taken into the HDL core.

In plasma, cholesterol ester transfer protein (CETP) is able to facilitate interchange of cholesterol ester and triglyceride between VLDL, HDL and LDL particles. As a result, where there are higher HDL levels in the plasma, removal of cholesterol from arterial walls is normally facilitated, limiting the risk of atherosclerosis.

It is now recognised that lipid-poor apo-A particles synthesised in the liver or gut are able to receive cholesterol from cholesterol-replete cells through a receptor (the ABCA-1 receptor) that is active in the liver and in macrophages. These particles, through activity of the enzyme LCAT, then become mature HDL particles. These HDL particles can also receive cholesterol from cholesterol-rich cells through a further receptor called SR-B1.

1.14 Are triglycerides atherogenic?

Triglycerides are often a major contributor to atherosclerosis. All lipoprotein particles carry a mixture of cholesterol, cholesterol ester, triglycerides and phospholipid. When plasma triglycerides are elevated, abnormal lipoprotein and lipid metabolism is evident, and the composition of lipoproteins is altered.

In the very rare inherited absence of the tissue enzyme lipoprotein lipase exceedingly high levels of plasma triglycerides occur because dietary chylomicrons and hepatic VLDLs are not metabolised. These are *not* particularly atherogenic, but pose a considerable risk for acute pancreatitis.

When VLDLs are overproduced or poorly cleared, they acquire extra cholesterol ester, and are catabolised poorly. In exchange for their cholesterol ester, LDLs acquire triglyceride from VLDLs, but then shrink in size as the triglyceride is hydrolysed by hepatic lipase. These small dense, triglyceride-rich LDLs are more atherogenic and enter the arterial subintimal space where they stimulate macrophage activation and foam cell formation.

In clinical terms, therefore, where both moderately elevated plasma cholesterol and triglycerides are present, particularly when HDL-cholesterol is low, then atherosclerotic risk is increased. This profile is sometimes called the atherogenic lipoprotein profile (ALP).

When triglycerides are raised there are often other associated risk factors such as hypertension, glucose intolerance or diabetes mellitus, hyperuricaemia with or without gout, obesity and especially central adiposity. These are the features of the insulin resistance syndrome (*see* Q 4.3 *and Box 1.1*).

1.15 What is the atherogenic lipoprotein phenotype?

The 'atherogenic lipid profile' is the pattern seen in a substantial portion of the population, where triglycerides and cholesterol are both moderately raised and there is an associated lower level of HDL-cholesterol. The risk of atheroma is partly from elevation of LDL-cholesterol, but also from raised triglycerides with a low HDL-cholesterol. In these circumstances there is exchange of cholesterol in LDLs and HDLs with triglyceride in VLDLs (and chylomicrons) so that the LDL (and HDL) quality is abnormal. This triglyceride-enriched LDL is less readily removed through the normal liver LDL receptors, more readily recognised by macrophages, and is more atherogenic than the LDL level itself might suggest.

These patients need active treatment, firstly to lower the LDL level, but may also need additional measures such as a fibrate to improve the triglycerides and to improve the quality of LDL-cholesterol.

For a particular level of LDL-cholesterol, there are also more LDL molecules present when there is an excess of small dense LDLs compared to normal LDLs, since there is substantially less cholesterol per molecule on the former than the latter, yet it is the number of LDL molecules that favours atherogenesis.

1.16 What is lipoprotein(a)?

Lipoprotein(a) – Lp(a) – is a large molecule in the blood, derived from many (variable numbers in different individuals) plasminogen-like fragment repeats attached to an LDL molecule. Because of its LDL and its

---

BOX 1.1 Metabolic syndrome: ATPIII*

The diagnosis is made when three or more of the following are present:
1. Waist:
   men >40 inches (>102 cm) or women >35 inches (>88 cm)
2. Serum triglycerides: ≥ 1.7 mmol/L
3. HDL-cholesterol: <1.0 (men) or <1.3 (women) mmol/L
4. Blood pressure: $\geq 130/\geq 85$ mmHg
5. Fasting glucose: ≥ 6.1 mmol/L

---

* Definition from the National Cholesterol Education Program, Adult Treatment Panel III (2001).[2]

links to the clotting system molecule, plasminogen, Lp(a) may contribute to atherogenesis from both components. When present in high levels in the blood, it contributes as an extra risk factor to the other classical risk factors that may be present. Lp(a) is largely inherited both in the number of plasminogen-like complexes in the molecule and also in the total amount in the blood, and so is not readily directly treatable.

If someone is known to have a high Lp(a) concentration, then the cardiovascular risk from that individual's classical risk factors is increased. Any calculated value for absolute risk of developing a first cardiovascular event should then be uprated and classical risk factors treated more energetically.

PATIENT QUESTIONS

1.17 What are lipids?

'Lipids' are fats: fats are substances that do not dissolve in water.

Some of these are fats that we would recognise, such as butter, margarines, cooking oils and animal fat, and are called 'triglycerides'. Some of the fat in our bodies comes from these dietary fats. However, at the end of every meal any spare foodstuffs that are surplus to immediate requirements (whether they come from sugars or starches, fats or proteins, or alcohol) are converted by the liver to triglycerides, circulate in the blood, and are laid down in our adipose (fat) tissue as the energy stores for the body.

One of the important 'lipids', or fats, is cholesterol, which is an essential part of the body. Cholesterol is a steroid, from which chemical pathway also come some of the fat-soluble vitamins, cortisol, and the sex hormones oestrogen and testosterone.

1.18 Why is cholesterol important?

Cholesterol is important because the outer membrane (envelope) of every cell, and the internal membranes which divide up cell structures, have cholesterol as an essential structural part. Fats in the membranes allow different molecules to be retained in or excluded from different parts of cells, so allowing the cell's specialised functions to operate. For example, complex fats (including cholesterol) form insulation around nerve fibres to allow the electrical and chemical messages in nerves to operate.

Other 'lipids' are complex compounds that have specialist roles and are part of cell structure. From cholesterol we make bile salts that are essential for food digestion, the sex hormones oestrogen and testosterone, and also the fat-soluble vitamins A, D and E. We need very little circulating cholesterol to make these essential compounds and even with exceedingly low blood levels these compounds are still made without difficulty.

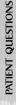

1.19   Where does cholesterol come from?

Some cholesterol comes into the body in the diet, and some is lost in the faeces. However, all cells in the body can make cholesterol, for it is an essential part of the outer 'envelope' or membranes of each cell, without which the cell could not exist or function. It is part of the 'bricks and mortar of the house'. In humans, most cells do not need to make cholesterol as the liver makes what is needed and this is delivered in the blood to all tissues throughout the body.

1.20   How much cholesterol do we need?

We need very little cholesterol in the diet. Diets for hyperlipidaemia suggest 200–300 mg per day of dietary cholesterol, and two or three egg yolks (being high in cholesterol) per week are sufficient. Most is made in the body by the liver and delivered to tissues that require it.

Too much cholesterol, and indeed too much dietary fat (triglycerides) – especially when saturated animal fat – tend to raise blood levels of cholesterol too high.

1.21   What is 'good' cholesterol?

So-called 'good' cholesterol is the cholesterol being carried on one of the blood particles called lipoproteins. This is called 'high density lipoprotein', usually abbreviated to HDL.

Cholesterol and blood fats cannot circulate 'loose' in the blood, which is a watery solution, as they would not dissolve. It would be a little like 'tepid lamb stew'! In order to circulate in the blood any fat or cholesterol absorbed in the gut, or any made and released from the liver has to circulate in large molecules in the blood where the fat is concealed in the middle. These are called lipoproteins, with the fats that are insoluble in water being inside an outer 'envelope' or membrane that has on the outside compounds that allow the whole particle to dissolve in water.

There are different types of lipoprotein that circulate in the blood that carry the fats and cholesterol. Some of these particles are taking cholesterol from the liver to other body tissues that require them, and some take cholesterol in the opposite direction.

The high density lipoprotein (HDL) particle is able to accept cholesterol from tissues in the body that have enough or too much. HDL particles take this cholesterol and carry it back to the liver for recycling ('the bus going back to the depot'). It is 'good' because the more HDL one has, the less cholesterol will tend to accumulate in the artery wall, which would otherwise encourage thickening and narrowing of the artery with heart attack and stroke risk.

1.22   What is 'bad' cholesterol?

Cholesterol that is made in the liver, including cholesterol absorbed from the diet that has initially gone to the liver, is carried around the body in a large molecule called 'low density lipoprotein', usually abbreviated to LDL.

This will supply cholesterol to all the tissues in the body that require it. It therefore has an essential role.

We only need quite low levels of circulating LDLs, and nearly all people have levels far above this low amount. The cholesterol on LDLs can become harmful, and hence the term 'bad' cholesterol, when there is too much circulating, for then it will gradually accumulate in the arteries of the body, leading to thickening and narrowing of these arteries and the later risk of heart attack and stroke.

Low density lipoprotein is therefore 'bad' only when there is too much circulating. Unfortunately, nearly all people have more than they need in the blood.

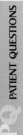

Atherosclerosis, lipids and cardiovascular disease

2

2.1	What are the risk factors that promote atherosclerosis?	18
2.2	How does an atherosclerotic plaque form?	18
2.3	What is a 'vulnerable' plaque?	19
2.4	What are the consequences of plaque rupture?	21
2.5	How common is atherosclerotic disease?	21
2.6	How strongly is cholesterol linked to atherosclerotic disease?	21
2.7	Is high cholesterol a risk factor for stroke?	22
2.8	What are normal levels of cholesterol?	24
2.9	What are normal levels of triglycerides?	27
2.10	How many people have high cholesterol?	27
2.11	Is low cholesterol safe?	27
2.12	Why do cholesterol levels differ between individuals?	28
2.13	Why do cholesterol levels differ between populations?	29
2.14	Why do some populations have lower rates of cardiovascular disease?	30
2.15	Why do some ethnic groups have higher rates of cardiovascular disease?	30
2.16	What is the importance of a family history of cardiovascular disease?	31

PQ PATIENT QUESTIONS

2.17	What is atherosclerosis?	33
2.18	What can happen to an atherosclerotic plaque?	33
2.19	What is cardiovascular disease?	34
2.20	How much do the major risk factors contribute to cardiovascular disease?	35

2.1 What are the risk factors that promote atherosclerosis?

There are fixed and modifiable risk factors. Atherosclerosis is a chronic inflammatory degenerative disease of the arterial wall, primarily affecting the endothelium and intima. Of fixed risk factors, age is therefore a primary factor in atherosclerosis as is the person's gender. The complex genetic background of an individual will contribute to their risk through multiple gene contributions currently only poorly understood, but there are also much better understood single gene disorders such as familial hypercholesterolaemia (*see Q 4.7*).

The classical major modifiable risk factors are hypercholesterolaemia, hypertension and smoking. Abnormal glucose control (diabetes mellitus and glucose intolerance) is a further risk factor independent of these. It is now recognised that 'hypercholesterolaemia' is insufficient as a description and lipid abnormalities can be re-defined as 'dyslipidaemia', for there are situations where other lipids or lipoproteins can be abnormal in quantity or quality. The main atherogenic lipoprotein abnormality is raised low density lipoprotein (LDL)-cholesterol (*see Q 1.12*). The lipid risk is increased when there are lower levels of high density lipoprotein (HDL)-cholesterol (*see Q 1.14*). Additionally, elevated levels of triglyceride-rich lipoproteins – very low density lipoproteins (VLDLs) (*see Qs 1.7 and 1.14*) and their remnants – are independently atherogenic.

Other factors also contribute to risk independently or through modification of other risks, but their influence is substantially less than for the classical risk factors. These may be inherited (e.g. lipoprotein(a); *see Q 1.16*) or environmentally influenced (e.g. blood homocysteine levels or obesity).

Elevated homocysteine levels are associated with excess coronary heart disease (CHD) risk and tend to be lower with higher folic acid levels, but as yet there are no long-term outcome studies of intervention on homocysteine levels (the SEARCH study of folic acid supplementation is due to report in 2005).

2.2 How does an atherosclerotic plaque form?

Recurrent, chronic damage occurs to the endothelium lining on the inside of the arterial wall through mechanical, toxic or biochemical effects. When damage occurs, a local inflammatory reaction results, and healing follows. Where risk factors are high, inflammation is accelerated and residual scarring accumulates.

The presence of LDL-cholesterol is an obligate for development of an atherosclerotic plaque.

In populations with low cholesterol levels such as Japan or China,[1,2] in the presence of hypertension or smoking cerebral haemorrhage and lung cancer are increased, but CHD rates remain relatively low. However. where Japanese populations move to other areas such as Hawaii and California and begin to take up the lifestyles to match, then their LDL levels and their CHD risks both rise.[2]

LDL-cholesterol enters the subintimal space undergoing minimal modification at the endothelium. Circulating blood monocytes are attracted to the endothelium at sites of damage, migrate between endothelial cells, and are immobilised and convert to macrophages in the subintimal space. These macrophages express receptors to take up modified or oxidised LDL and in the presence of high LDL levels become the foam cells of the fatty streak. They also lead to expression of monocyte-attractant molecules on the plasma membrane to further increase the entry of these white cells into the artery's subintimal space. At the same time, smooth muscle cells move from the media of the artery into the subintimal space. Here they produce collagen, glycosaminoglycans and matrix components, the ground substance of the fatty streak.

Most of these areas of minor arterial wall damage heal fully, but in some the residual tissue leads to thickened areas and plaque. As this occurs, there is remodelling of the artery that expands a little, largely preserving the lumen of the vessel. Only as recurrent damage, lipid deposition and scarring occur does the plaque expand to narrow the vessel. The endothelium over the plaque may become acutely breached, leading to platelet aggregation and local thrombosis. In many instances this thrombotic area heals and is incorporated into the plaque, perhaps with narrowing of the vessel lumen, but only rarely does the vessel occlude from this thrombosis (*Fig. 2.1*). Angiography therefore does not demonstrate the extent of atherosclerosis, most of the lesions not being demonstrated due to this remodelling. Most lesions in the arterial wall are therefore silent, and it is only the advanced lesions that narrow the artery and give rise to symptoms of angina. It is often the silent lesions which suddenly worsen that give rise to acute thrombosis and myocardial infarction. Lesions that are more likely to do this are termed 'vulnerable plaques' (*see* Q 2.3).

2.3   What is a 'vulnerable' plaque?

A vulnerable plaque is a plaque where there is a higher rate of inflammation. These plaques have more macrophages and foam cells, but fewer smooth muscle cells forming a fibrous cap over the lesion. Damage occurs at susceptible areas of an arterial wall (e.g. at arterial bifurcations) and leads to an inflammatory response as part of a potentially healing process.

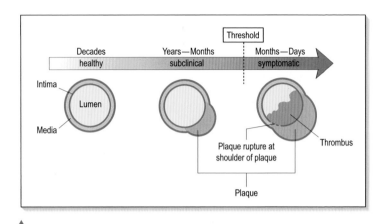

▲

Fig. 2.1 Atherogenesis is an inflammatory and degenerative process affecting the arterial wall over years and decades. Recurrent minor damage to the arterial wall occurs from high cholesterol and blood fats, from high blood pressure, use of tobacco products, and from diabetes. This leads to lipid deposition in the subintimal space and ingress of monocytes transforming into macrophages to take up lipid and apoptotic cell products. Smooth muscle cells from the arterial media also enter the subintimal space to provide collagen and matrix components. There are features of inflammation, healing and scarring with cytokines and vasoactive substances produced. Initial damage is healed, but local thrombosis can occur and atheromatous plaques develop. As this occurs, the arterial wall remodels to maintain a (near)-normal vessel lumen. Only when very extensive plaques develop, and endothelial breaches lead to platelet thrombus, does the vessel lumen begin to narrow critically. (Adapted from Ross.[3])

After endothelial damage, LDL molecules enter the subintimal space; monocytes are also attracted there from the blood being immobilised and transformed into macrophages. The macrophages take up LDL (particularly modified LDL molecules) to become foam cells. Meanwhile smooth muscle cells enter from the media and lay down collagen and glycosaminoglycans as the matrix of the plaque, and form a fibrous cap over the lesion. Where there is a relative excess of macrophages or foam cells over smooth muscle cells the plaque becomes more vulnerable and has a thinner overlying fibrous cap separating it from the vessel lumen. The fat-loaded macrophages make their way out of the plaque through the fibrous cap. They release metalloproteinases which break down the fibrous cap. Plaques with thin caps are much more likely to rupture at their shoulders. These vulnerable plaques contain relatively more lipid. Lowering blood LDL levels reduces the amount of cholesterol and lipid that enters the plaque, and over time leads to stabilisation of these more vulnerable plaques.

2.4   What are the consequences of plaque rupture?

When there is rupture of a plaque, cytokines and vasoactive compounds are released. These lead to rapid activation of platelets that adhere to the lesion and form a plug.

Many of these acute episodes are self-limiting, the platelets sealing the ruptured area, scar tissue being formed and, over time, the lesion heals. The plaque may gradually enlarge, but rather than narrowing the artery significantly, the artery remodels to a somewhat larger overall size so that the lumen is not greatly reduced.

With multiple such episodes, a plaque of substantial size may develop, often with calcification, leading to major vessel narrowing and (in the coronary arteries) to exercise-induced myocardial ischaemia and angina pectoris.

However, in some episodes of plaque rupture, the platelet aggregation and thrombus that forms is not limited and rapidly extends, leading to vessel occlusion. Distal to the vessel occlusion acute ischaemia and tissue necrosis occur, with myocardial infarction and stroke as potential consequences.

2.5   How common is atherosclerotic disease?

Atherosclerotic disease – commonly cardiac, cerebral, renal or peripheral vascular – is the commonest cause of death in the westernised world (*Fig. 2.2*). Around a quarter of a million macrovascular deaths occur in the UK per year.

In the UK, of every myocardial infarction, about 30% are fatal. In the other 70% of individuals, the subsequent life expectancy is approximately halved compared to an unaffected individual, and the quality of that remaining life expectancy may be reduced by further events (e.g. angina, cardiac failure, etc.).

Rates are increased in those with diabetes mellitus, those of Asian origin or those with inherited conditions such as familial hypercholesterolaemia (*see Q 4.7*). Rates are increased in relation to the classical risk factors of smoking, hypertension and hypercholesterolaemia (dyslipidaemia; *see Q 4.1*). Central adiposity and insulin resistance are further links.

2.6   How strongly is cholesterol linked to atherosclerotic disease?

High cholesterol, hypertension, smoking and diabetes are the classical risk factors predisposing to atherosclerotic macrovascular disease. Of these, high cholesterol is a near obligate, for vascular disease is at very low rates in

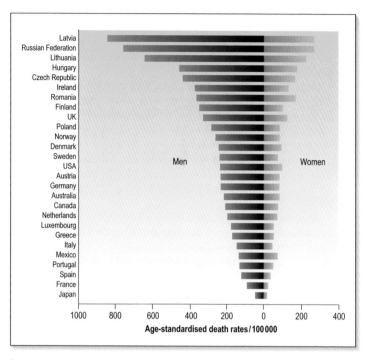

Fig. 2.2 Comparison of death rates from coronary heart disease, men and women, aged 35–74, in different westernised countries. Based on data from the World Health Organization (www.who.int/en)

populations such as the rural Chinese[1] and Japanese where cholesterol levels are low, even though hypertension and smoking may be prevalent.

The relationship between blood cholesterol levels and macrovascular risk has been demonstrated in many studies, across different countries (*Fig. 2.3*) and in single countries in large studies such as over several decades in the Framingham study (*Fig. 2.4*) or in over a third of a million men in the MRFIT study (*Fig. 2.5*).[6–8]

2.7 Is high cholesterol a risk factor for stroke?

High cholesterol is a risk factor for all forms of macrovascular disease. In epidemiological studies, such as the Framingham study, there is a clear relationship between cholesterol and stroke and cerebrovascular disease. The relationship between rising cholesterol and stroke risk is not as strong

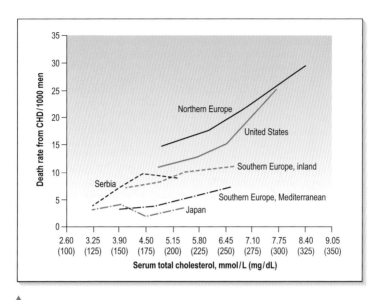

Fig. 2.3 The progressive increase in mortality from coronary heart disease risk as serum total cholesterol rises is seen in various countries with different absolute risk of disease – The Seven Countries Study. (After Verschuren et al.[4])

as that with CHD. This relationship is primarily with atherosclerotic, thrombotic stroke and not with haemorrhagic stroke.

It has been of particular interest, and beneficial to patients, that when cholesterol and LDL-cholesterol levels are lowered the reduction in stroke is substantial and significantly greater than might be expected from the epidemiological evidence. This means that the reductions in stroke rates in the major statin randomised controlled trials (RCTs) have been of about the same percentage as the reductions in CHD rates. On an intention-to-treat basis the reductions have been around 25–50%. The reductions are potentially greater on an 'on-treatment' basis, and greater where more substantial LDL-cholesterol reductions are achieved.

The new Joint British Societies' guideline charts[9] identify cardiovascular (CHD and stroke) risk and advise treatment for primary prevention at ≥20% 10-year risk. The older 15% and 30% 10-year CHD risks correspond to 20% and 40% 10-year cardiovascular risk.

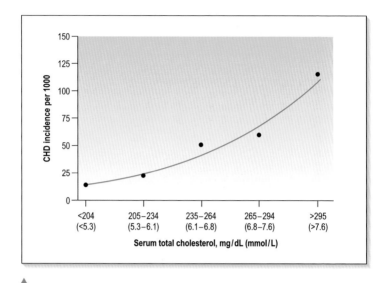

Fig. 2.4 The relationship between increasing coronary heart disease (CHD) risk as LDL-cholesterol rises in the Framingham population. The incidence of CHD rises in a semi-log linear manner over a wide range of cholesterol levels. Studies in other populations have shown that the same relationship applies, at different levels of absolute risk, and that the relationship extends to much lower total cholesterol levels as seen in Chinese populations. (From Castelli,[5] with permission from Excerpta Medica, Inc.)

2.8 What are normal levels of cholesterol?

There is a broad spread of cholesterol and triglyceride levels in the population; additionally, levels vary across different countries.

'Normal' levels can be defined in relation to the overall levels in the population, usually as the 95% confidence interval (mean ± 2 SD). This would place 2.5% of the population as having 'abnormal' low and another 2.5% as having 'abnormal' high levels. This definition does not reflect the clinical relevance of the cholesterol or triglyceride, and really defines 'usual' rather than normal levels.

In the UK the mean cholesterol in adults is around 5.6 mmol/L (*Table 2.1*), and triglycerides about 1.4 mmol/L. Values of cholesterol are lower by around 1.0–1.5 mmol/L in childhood, rising after puberty. Cholesterol values are fairly similar in males and females, although in women there are higher HDL-cholesterol levels contributing to the total cholesterol. In women, cholesterol and LDL-cholesterol levels tend to rise after the menopause, and the mean level is then a little higher than in men.

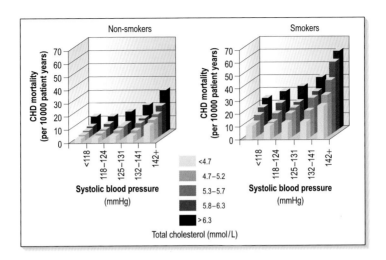

Fig. 2.5 Coronary heart disease mortality in 356 000 middle-aged men in the USA in relation to smoking habit and systolic blood pressure. (Based on data from Stamler et al.[8])

TABLE 2.1 Mean serum cholesterol levels in England 1998		
Age (years)	Men	Women
16–24	4.4	4.6
25–34	5.1	4.9
35–44	5.5	5.2
45–54	5.8	5.7
55–64	5.8	6.2
65–74	5.8	6.4
75+	5.5	6.3
All	5.5	5.6

The levels of cholesterol and LDL-cholesterol in humans are maintained at substantially higher levels than are essential for health, even in communities that have relatively low mean values such as in Japan or China[1] (*see Fig. 2.4*). Babies have LDL-cholesterol levels of 1 mmol/L or less without interfering with development.

Perhaps 'normal' cholesterol levels should be defined as those at which health maintenance is optimal and illness minimised. In epidemiological studies within and across communities there is a continuous relationship for cholesterol against both cardiovascular and total mortality. We are aware of the low rates of heart disease in hunter–gatherer and subsistence farming cultures, where levels of cholesterol are low and perhaps these societies offer the best definition of 'normal' cholesterol (*Table 2.2*). Even at mean levels of 3.5 mmol/L, because cholesterol levels are continuously related to heart disease, some CHD events will still occur.

The relationship follows a semi-log-linear pattern, without evidence for a cholesterol level below which there is no further potential benefit, and without evidence of harm. In the major intervention trials, usually of several thousand patients over a period of 3–6 years (using alone, or in combination, diet, lifestyle, statins, other drugs, ileal bypass), the achieved reductions in cholesterol and LDL-cholesterol have shown benefits in cardiovascular risk and, in studies and meta-analyses in total mortality, down to low lipid levels. Several studies (HPS,[10] ASCOT-LLA,[11] GREACE,[12] LIPS,[13] CARDS[14]) have reduced mean LDL-cholesterol well below 3 mmol/L and with the same relative risk reduction whether initial LDL values were higher or lower, there being benefit to well below 2 mmol/L. Recently PROVE-IT[15] and TNT[16] have shown extra benefit when LDL-cholesterol levels were reduced to a mean of 1.6 mmol/L compared to 2.5 mmol/L, and 2.0 mmol/L compared to 2.6 mmol/L, respectively.

These data suggest that almost all in the population run lipid levels higher than desirable, and populations will benefit by measures that reduce mean lipid levels in communities. For all people adoption of healthy diet, exercise and lifestyle measures are sensible, while individuals at higher cardiovascular risk may need additional measures, including drug therapy. However, it will not be the absolute level alone that will indicate the need for pharmacological intervention, but the absolute risk that an individual has because of the integrated risk from all environmental and inherited factors, and the intervention(s) will need to tackle all elevated or abnormal levels.

TABLE 2.2 Typical cholesterol values in men aged 45–64 years in different populations

	Population	Cholesterol (mmol/L)
	Hunter–gatherer societies	3–3.5
Increasing CHD prevalence	Rural China	3.5
	Rural Japan	4.5
	Urban Japan	5.0
	Mediterranean countries	5.2–5.6
	USA	5.7
	Northern Europe	6–6.4
	Finland 1980	7.0

2.9   What are normal levels of triglycerides?

High levels of triglycerides tend to be associated with lower levels of the 'protective' HDL-cholesterol and increased risk. When triglycerides are 1.5–5.0 mmol/L, some triglyceride exchanges into LDL and HDL. This triglyceride is removed in the liver, and the resultant 'small dense' LDL is significantly more atherogenic.

When triglycerides are very high – ≥10 mmol/L (and cholesterol levels tend to be pulled up by about 1 mmol/L for every 5 mmol/L of triglyceride elevation) – the risk is less of cardiovascular disease (CVD) but more of acute pancreatitis when different considerations apply (but treatment is needed).

2.10   How many people have high cholesterol?

Cholesterol values in the adult population average 5.6 mmol/L. About 70% of the untreated population have total cholesterol levels above 5 mmol/L, and perhaps 90% have levels above 4 mmol/L, below which is the target for people at significantly increased cardiovascular disease risk. Most of the population would benefit from simple diet, weight loss, exercise and lifestyle measures to minimise their cholesterol and lipid levels, and there is no evidence to suggest that individuals would be at any increased risk from following a healthy prudent lifestyle.
Clearly 90% of the population do not warrant pharmacotherapy!

2.11   Is low cholesterol safe?

Around 10–20 years ago suggestions were made that low cholesterol levels put individuals at risk of other disease. These were false or erroneous interpretations of the data and have been refuted.

It was suggested that individuals with low cholesterol levels had increased malignancy risk, but this is not the same as saying that reducing cholesterol to low levels causes malignancy. In the 356 000 middle aged men followed, but not treated, as screenees from the Multiple Risk Factor Intervention Trial (MRFIT),[6–8] malignancy such as carcinoma of the colon was increased at low cholesterol levels. However, the excess malignancy almost always occurred in the first year or so of follow-up, and not thereafter in up to 14 years of follow-up. These individuals would have had their malignancy, known or still occult, at entry into the study, and as with other catabolic states, the cholesterol would have fallen somewhat (as it does for example with intentional weight loss).

The other 'risks' suggested were that patients with low cholesterol levels would be more violent or have increased suicide rates, following small number differences in the Lipid Research Clinics – Coronary Primary Prevention Trial (LRC-CPPT) with colestyramine and the Helsinki Heart Study with gemfibrozil. However, the violence in the colestyramine trial was not that individuals became violent but had violence done unto them by chance. These events and the small excess of suicides in the gemfibrozil study were examined in detail by the US Food and Drug Administration (www.fda.gov) and were not found to be related to medication.

In more recent studies, where the more efficacious statin drugs have been used, there has been no evidence to suggest these problems are increased and no significant differences have been found in adverse events between the placebo and verum groups. This has been in groups with quite widely different LDL-cholesterol levels. Recent studies[10–15] have lowered LDL-cholesterol very substantially to 2.5 mmol/L and below. In the Heart Protection Study[10] the lowest tercile of patients had their LDL-cholesterol lowered to 1.8 mmol/L and in the recent PROVE-IT study[15] the more actively treated group had a mean LDL-cholesterol over 4 years of 1.6 mmol/L, with a further 16% reduction in cardiovascular risk compared to the less actively treated group at 2.5 mmol/L. TNT[16] also showed that achieving low levels of LDL-cholesterol was both beneficial and safe.

It may be of interest to recognise that babies and infants have an LDL-cholesterol of 1 mmol/L or less, without detriment to physical or mental development.

2.12 Why do cholesterol levels differ between individuals?

There are random, methodological, inherited and environmental reasons for cholesterol variation.

RANDOM

In an individual with no overt reason for variation, the cholesterol will vary above and below a 'true' value. The coefficient of variation for such variation is ± 6%, so the 95% confidence levels for a single value will be ± 12%. Thus in an individual whose 'true' cholesterol value is, for example, 6 mmol/L, on this basis a single value could be between 5.3 and 6.7 mmol/L by chance with 2.5% of values being above and 2.5% being below this range. When two or more sample values are averaged this potential variation is substantially reduced. This does need to be borne in mind when assessing both a patient's risk and response to treatment.

METHODOLOGICAL

A further such variation will also occur in the laboratory, but in central NHS laboratories in the UK, with external standardisation and quality control this variation will be 2% or less. Using pharmacy testing some methods can be just as good depending on the user, but some methods (and especially some of the stick tests) can have very wide variation and are not recommended.

INHERITED

Some individuals will have genetic factors contributing to their high or low cholesterol levels. These may be single gene disorders such as in familial hypercholesterolaemia (*see* Q 4.7) where affected heterozygous individuals may have doubling of their cholesterol levels. In other disorders such as familial dysbetalipoproteinaemia (remnant lipaemia, type III hyperlipidaemia; *see* Q 2.16) while 1% of the population has the genetic disorder very few become hyperlipidaemic. Indeed, many of these patients have very slightly lower LDL-cholesterol values. However, in about 2% of those affected the presence of another genetic contribution or commonly a significant environmental factor leads to accumulation of remnant lipoproteins that are not rapidly catabolised. Here both cholesterol and triglycerides rise, often to values for both in the range of 6–12 mmol/L.

In many individuals there will be small contributions from the effects of multiple genes that contribute to particular high or low lipid levels, although many of these genetic contributors have not been delineated.

ENVIRONMENTAL

Secondary or environmental causes include disease states and lifestyle factors. Disorders such as diabetes, renal and hepatic disease and hypothyroidism will alter lipid levels and need to be excluded and/or considered in lipid management. Individuals who are sedentary and in those with overweight or obesity (particularly central adiposity) lipid abnormalities increase, and are more likely to be a mixed hyperlipidaemia or dyslipidaemia with raised triglycerides and low HDL-cholesterol. Within populations there can also be some drift in lipid levels reflecting dietary, weight and exercise variation with the seasons. In most individuals this will not be of a magnitude to be personally identified.

2.13 Why do cholesterol levels differ between populations?

There can be wide variations between populations, on a nation basis, or in groups within a country's population. An early study was that of Ancel Keys[17] in the Seven Countries Study (*see* Fig. 2.3). Japanese and especially rural Chinese populations[1] have low cholesterol levels, but in their urban populations levels are higher. Much of this is environmental rather than genetic/racial. Where Japanese populations have migrated eastward from Japan to Hawaii and on to California, to an extent that they take up the lifestyle to match, they acquire the cholesterol values and the cardiovascular risk of the population of the adopted country.[2] This is also seen as an issue in the South Asian population who, on taking up westernised lifestyles, develop significant mixed dyslipidaemia with features of the insulin resistance syndrome (*see Q 4.3 and Box 1.1*) and premature macrovascular disease.[18]

2.14 Why do some populations have lower rates of cardiovascular disease?

Lower rates of cardiovascular disease in different populations can usually be substantially explained by the prevalence of the known major risk factors of smoking, hypertension, hyperlipidaemia/dyslipidaemia and diabetes.

Some populations have more lipid-friendly diets and in the presence of lower cholesterol levels the Japanese, for example, have low CHD rates, even though they have high rates of smoking, hypertension and stroke.

Cholesterol and LDL-cholesterol have a 'facilitatory' role, and if LDL-cholesterol levels are sufficiently low, then other risk factors have much more limited effect.

Environmental factors also have substantial roles in hyperlipidaemia and dyslipidaemia. As populations see major increases in overweight and obesity there are accompanying increases in lipid values, often with hypertriglyceridaemia and low HDL-cholesterol levels.

Dietary variations may contribute to the differences between the southern European and northern European populations. Higher HDL-cholesterol levels are likely to account for at least some of the relative protection of premenopausal females compared to males. Different rates of smoking in males and females will contribute to some of the gender differences, but in some female populations where smoking rates have increased over recent decades, CHD rates will be expected to follow. In France, smoking rates were lower in the initial decades after the Second World War than, for example, in the UK, but subsequently increased.

2.15 Why do some ethnic groups have higher rates of cardiovascular disease?

It is clear that the rates of cardiovascular disease are substantially higher in Southern Asian populations when they follow a more westernised lifestyle. This is true whether in the UK, or when one compares other countries, such as in Fiji, when Fijian and Asian communities are compared whether urbanised or more rural. Other communities such as the Micronesians and some American Indians also have increased rates.

How much of this may be genetic is uncertain. When generations have lived in situations where intermittent natural disaster or famine occurs it is possible that those with a 'thrifty gene' background have survival benefit. However, where exercise profiles reduce and food is less limited, then increased adiposity (with diabetes following) may have detrimental effects.

Certainly, in Indian subcontinent populations there are higher rates of the insulin resistance syndrome (*see* Q 4.3 *and Box 1.1*) with abdominal obesity, mixed hyperlipidaemia, hypertension, glucose intolerance or diabetes, hyperuricaemia and gout. These are associated with accelerated atherogenesis. In Japanese and Chinese populations, cholesterol levels and CHD rates are quite low but cerebrovascular disease is higher related to blood pressure and perhaps salt intake. Japanese diabetes rates are high, and CHD and CVD rates are rising, likely to be partly related to changes in lifestyle.

2.16 What is the importance of a family history of cardiovascular disease?

Family history is an important contributor to cardiovascular risk, and is not always fully assessed and incorporated into an individual's risk calculation. CVD risk relates to the interaction between an individual's genetic background and the environmental factors operating.

ASSESSING THE GENETIC CONTRIBUTION

Some individuals will inherit single gene disorders giving rise to cardiovascular disease, but in many in the population there will be contributions from multiple genes that are currently poorly understood. Clinically, the genetic contribution should be assessed by enquiry of family history, of the presence of macrovascular disease in parents together with its nature, age of initial onset and presence of known risk factors. Age of onset in first degree male relatives before the age of 55, and in females before 65 years, is clearly likely to be of importance. Enquiry should also be made of uncles, aunts, siblings and children. Taking into account the number of such relatives, the greater the number and the earlier the age of onset of disease provides some guide to the genetic component and to the risk. The guidelines of the Joint British Societies (published on the web at the BMJ March 2004) (http://bmj.bmjjournals.com/cgi/content/full/320/7236/705) suggest that the calculated risk should be augmented by 50%, but this is likely to be an underestimate in some more severely affected families.

SPECIFIC SINGLE GENE DISORDERS

Where specific single gene disorders are encountered in a family, then this is of major significance, and it may well be possible to identify at-risk members of that family. The classic example is familial hypercholesterolaemia (*see* Q 4.7) affecting 1 in 500 of the population in the heterozygous form, and 1 in 1 000 000 in the homozygous form. The gene defect can be identified in around 50–75% of those affected, but as there are more than 700 known defects in the gene it may not be that straightforward, unless a defect has already been found in another family member. Finding the gene defect does not currently influence treatment. Where one person has been found to have familial hypercholesterolaemia, then one parent is an obligate heterozygote, and each sibling and child has a 50% risk.

A further rare condition is familial dysbetalipoproteinaemia (remnant lipaemia, type III hyperlipidaemia) where there is homozygosity for the E2 pattern of apolipoprotein E. About 1% of the population has this, but only about 2% of these then develop severe mixed hyperlipidaemia, nearly always when there is at least one other disease, environmental or inherited factor. Here premature CHD and peripheral vascular disease can present at a very early age but the hyperlipidaemia and the risk respond well to diet and weight loss treatment, and if necessary to fibrate treatment. Fibrates are the drug group of first choice, but statins can be helpful, and in a few patients a statin-fibrate (usually with fenofibrate, and *not* gemfibrozil) is needed (*see Ch. 7*). Other siblings and members of the family may also be affected. A fibrate drug may be the drug of choice (a statin being second line) in individuals with remnant lipaemia inadequately responding to diet and lifestyle change.

SCREENING FAMILY MEMBERS

Whether there is a clear single gene disorder or a possible polygenic contribution to a family history of vascular disease, it is of considerable importance to ensure that other first degree members of the family are screened (and any second degree relatives where a further family member is found with hyperlipidaemia). These relatives are often not patients of the proband's doctor, and the proband needs to be strongly encouraged to contact all the family to obtain lipid profiles.

In 2004, the UK Department of Health agreed to initiate a cascade screening programme, where specially trained nurses in the community would contact the first degree relatives of patients with familial hypercholesterolaemia to check their profiles, since 50% of these individuals will also be affected. Where such an individual is so affected, their relatives in turn will be approached. It is hoped that the pilot studies that began in the autumn of 2004 will be the prelude to a national roll-out, for only 10–15% of affected individuals are currently identified. This will be a clinically based programme, but a similar programme is already in operation in Holland, although with the underlying LDL receptor genetic defect also being sought.

PATIENT QUESTIONS

2.17   What is atherosclerosis?

Atherosclerosis is the name given to disease of the main arteries in the body, where these are gradually damaged over many years. The lining of the artery is damaged by a number of factors, of which the main ones are high blood pressure, tobacco use, high blood fats and cholesterol, and diabetes. Parts of the smooth inner lining of the artery have repeated minor damage, get inflamed and then heal with some scarring. Much of the time the local injury heals, but over time more severe changes occur. One can imagine the process to be akin to recurrent minor injuries to the skin.

Some areas of the arteries are more vulnerable than others, such as where the flow of blood is more turbulent where an artery branches. With scarring, some thickening of the wall of an artery occurs. While the artery initially maintains its inner size, gradually it becomes narrowed and the flow of blood is restricted. Where heart arteries are narrowed, not enough blood is provided to give sufficient oxygen to the heart muscle at times of increased exercise. This leads to the chest pain on exertion that is called angina (*see* Q 2.19).

These thickened and narrowed areas of the arteries accumulate cholesterol and fat. When blood cholesterol is high, more fat accumulates, and these areas are vulnerable to acute deterioration. When this occurs the thin inner lining of the artery (the endothelium) is damaged. Blood platelets rapidly stick together over the damaged lining. When we sustain a cut this process seals the bleeding, but on the inside of the artery a blood clot or thrombosis may partly or completely block the artery. Where this occurs in the heart, the heart muscle served by that artery can die, and this is the process of 'heart attack' that follows this 'coronary thrombosis'. The same process in the brain is a 'cerebral thrombosis' leading to a 'stroke'.

The process of atherosclerosis is a gradual degenerative or 'ageing' process over decades, which can then lead to sudden acute illness or death, but which can be accelerated or delayed depending on risk factor changes.

2.18   What can happen to an atherosclerotic plaque?

An atherosclerotic plaque is a local area of damage to an artery, where there is thickening in the wall of the artery. The plaque contains fat and cholesterol, and may accumulate chalk. Often this will not narrow the inside of the artery nor affect the flow of blood, unless a very major plaque has formed.

The inflammation within the plaque can sometimes be greater than the scarring or healing process. This is more likely in plaques that contain a lot of fat (cholesterol and triglyceride). Then the thin inner lining of the artery (the endothelium) suffers a break in its surface. The chemicals released lead to rapid sticking of platelets over the surface to seal this break. With the platelets a blood clot (a thrombosis) forms which narrows the artery. This process is going on within our arteries, unknowingly to us, on a regular basis.

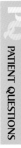

PATIENT QUESTIONS

If we are lucky, then the thrombosis only partially blocks the artery. Then gradually this clot is absorbed, incorporated into the artery, and a new inner surface lining is formed. Healing has occurred, but the artery may have become rather more narrowed than before, and repeats of such processes will continue to narrow the artery until blood flow is restricted and symptoms occur (e.g. angina, intermittent claudication; *see Q 2.19*). If we are unlucky, then the thrombosis extends to the whole artery that is then blocked, leading to a sudden stroke or heart attack.

2.19   What is cardiovascular disease?

Cardiovascular disease refers to disorders of the heart and circulatory system. Most of these refer to the processes of damage, narrowing and blocking of the arteries by atherosclerosis (*see Qs 2.2 and 2.17*). The clinical results can affect any of the principal arteries of the main trunk (the aorta) leading from the heart, such as the branches that feed blood to the heart itself (coronary arteries), to the brain (cerebral arteries), to the gut and bowel, to the legs, and indeed to all organs. The main consequences are heart attack and angina, stroke and poor blood circulation affecting brain function, and pain in leg muscles limiting ability to walk. Other symptoms can occur depending on the artery and organ affected.

As the arteries (the coronary arteries) that feed the heart muscle get narrowed, when a person then takes exercise and the heart muscle has to work harder, insufficient blood is supplied to the heart. With insufficient oxygen and waste chemical substances not being removed, muscle pain results. This is the tightening, constricting pain or discomfort in the front of the chest (and which may spread to (usually left) shoulder and upper arm) that is called angina. When the person rests, the pain then subsides as normal oxygen supply is enough for the resting heart muscle.

When a coronary artery blocks, then the heart muscle beyond the block has acute blood and oxygen shortage; this results in damage to the heart and some people will die. This is the acute coronary (artery) thrombosis leading to the acute heart attack. Nowadays, with emergency drug treatment to break up the blood clot in the coronary artery it is possible to limit substantially the size of the heart attack and how much muscle dies. In some hospitals it may also be possible to do emergency heart artery X-rays (an angiogram) and open up the acute blockage of the artery (an angioplasty).

Blockage of an artery going to the brain is called a cerebral thrombosis and leads to permanent brain damage – a stroke. Narrowing of leg arteries limits blood flow to leg muscles, and discomfort and pain in the muscles (usually of the calf) limits walking ability, this being termed 'intermittent claudication'. If a leg artery blocks acutely then there is a risk of gangrene of the extremities. If this block cannot be opened up with an angioplasty or surgically bypassed, there is then an amputation risk.

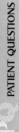

PATIENT QUESTIONS

2.20 How much do the major risk factors contribute to cardiovascular disease?

There are a large number of possible risk factors for cardiovascular disease (coronary heart disease and stroke), some of which are fixed and some of which are alterable. The major risk factors that are fixed and not alterable are gender (risks in males being higher than in females), increasing age and genetic predisposition. The main modifiable risk factors that account for most of the alterable risk are cholesterol and blood fats levels, high blood pressure, tobacco use and diabetes.

High blood pressure puts extra strain on the arteries and damages the inner lining of the artery – the 'endothelium'. Tobacco use also causes this type of damage. When there is damage then inflammation in the artery wall occurs (a little like the inflammation that may occur temporarily when we damage our skin which then heals over in a few days or so). High cholesterol levels get into the artery wall, especially where there is surface damage to the endothelium. The more cholesterol there is in the artery wall the greater the degree of inflammation. This inflammation can then lead to local scarring, and over months and decades this can gradually narrow the artery.

Diabetes also contributes by altering metabolism in the artery wall. Even allowing for factors such as blood pressure, cholesterol and tobacco, diabetes in its own right at any age increases the risk two to three times in males, and three to four times in females.

Measuring lipids

3

3.1	Who should have their lipids measured?	38
3.2	Where should lipid testing take place?	38
3.3	What tests should be done?	39
3.4	How is LDL-cholesterol measured?	40
3.5	What abnormalities of lipids are seen?	40
3.6	How accurate are the measurements?	41
3.7	How do lipid levels change according to age and gender?	43
3.8	How often should lipid tests be repeated?	43

PQ PATIENT QUESTIONS

3.9	What is 'the lipid profile'?	44
3.10	How would I know if my lipid profile was abnormal?	45
3.11	What levels are desirable?	45

3.1 Who should have their lipids measured?

The National Cholesterol Education Program (NCEP) in the USA recommends cholesterol screening for all adults over the age of 20.[1] The argument is that empowering individuals with knowledge about their lipid profile provides an incentive for change but this has not been proved and the information may even encourage less healthy behaviour if the results are reassuring.

Other authorities have recommended the abandonment of lipid testing altogether in favour of treating high cardiovascular risk, citing the results of the Heart Protection Study (HPS) which underlined the benefit of lipid-lowering treatment for individuals at high cardiovascular risk irrespective of their baseline lipid levels. The problem with this approach is that certain high-risk individuals (e.g. those with familial hyperlipidaemia) are often unidentified and both they and undiagnosed family members may miss out on treatment. In addition, all practitioners are familiar with the interest shown by patients in their test results and this can potentially be harnessed as an important factor in compliance with subsequent treatment.

A compromise approach is to offer lipid testing selectively to those whose cardiovascular risk profile suggests they have most to gain by the extra information (*Box 3.1*).

3.2 Where should lipid testing take place?

The development of the primary care team with its multidisciplinary, patient-centred approach lends itself to individual cardiovascular risk factor assessment and primary care doctors and nurses are becoming increasingly

---

BOX 3.1 Patients with a high cardiovascular risk profile

Such patients include those:

- with a personal history of CHD, PAD or cerebrovascular disease (for secondary prevention)
- with a family history of CHD or PAD (especially before age 55 years) or hyperlipidaemia
- with hypertension
- with diabetes mellitus
- with physical stigmata of hyperlipidaemia
- with obesity (BMI >30)
- with chronic renal disease
- who smoke.

CHD, coronary heart disease; PAD, peripheral arterial disease.

skilled in assessing the implications of abnormal lipid levels. The task of primary cardiovascular disease prevention is, however, enormous and constrained in primary care by the lack of human resources and the drive of current initiatives to focus on secondary prevention. The advent of portable dry chemistry devices has enabled more widespread testing and lipid testing is now available from a number of providers including pharmacists and commercial organisations. From the perspective of clinical governance, wherever lipid testing is undertaken, there need to be quality assurances about the accuracy of risk factor estimation and assessment, the quality of counselling and advice given and appropriate liaison with the patient and conventional medical services.

3.3 What tests should be done?

Data from the British Regional Heart Study show that knowledge of serum cholesterol alone fails to distinguish clearly between the population that suffers from coronary heart disease (CHD) and the population that does not. Clearly, this is due to the interactive influence of the other cardiovascular risk factors and the more information that is available regarding an individual's risk profile, the more accurate the assessment of risk. As far as lipids are concerned, trying to interpret their influence on risk based on a total cholesterol result is akin to trying to evaluate anaemia without access to measures of red cell morphology or haematinics.

> Fasting has little effect on total serum cholesterol and high density lipoprotein (HDL) cholesterol levels. In general population screening, where triglyceride estimation is unnecessary, non-fasting specimens are adequate and this makes the test more acceptable to patients. Triglyceride levels are affected by meals and in healthy subjects it takes up to 8 hours to produce a steady triglyceride level. A reasonable approach, as suggested by the NCEP, is detailed in *Box 3.2*.

Apolipoprotein B (apo-B) is found not only in low density lipoprotein (LDL) but also in very low density lipoprotein (VLDL) and remnant particles, and as such represents a truer reflection of the burden of atherogenic particles. Large studies such as AMORIS and the Quebec Heart Study suggest the increased predictive power of apolipoprotein measurements including apo-B, apo-AI and the ratio of apo-B to apo-AI. Ongoing surveys, such as the recent INTERHEART case-control study (*see* Q 5.5), will define whether or not the additional measurement of apolipoproteins enables superior risk categorisation over conventional parameters.[2]

> **BOX 3.2 National Cholesterol Education Program lipid screening in adults**
>
> ■ Age:
>   — ≥20 years
> ■ Appropriate screening:
>   — universal
>   — opportunistic
> ■ Non-fasting TC and HDL-cholesterol in:
>   — healthy individuals
>   — fasting lipid profile if high TC, low HDL-cholesterol or borderline
>   high TC + ≥ two other risk factors
> ■ Full fasting profile where:
>   — atherosclerosis present
>   — diabetes present
>   — high multiple risk
>   — physician chooses
>
> HDL, high density lipoprotein; TC, total cholesterol.

3.4 How is LDL-cholesterol measured?

Although LDL-cholesterol is the major therapeutic target in most patients, its value is usually determined by calculation from the other elements of the fasting lipid profile.

LDL-cholesterol is derived using the Friedewald formula,[3] where all measurements are in mmol/L:

$$\text{LDL-cholesterol} = \text{total cholesterol} - \text{HDL-cholesterol} - \text{total triglycerides}/2.19.$$

The function – total triglycerides/2.19 – provides an estimate of VLDL-cholesterol and is reasonably accurate up to triglyceride values of 4.5 mmol/L. Beyond this, direct LDL-cholesterol measurement is required.

LDL-cholesterol can be measured directly but the reagents are relatively expensive compared to using the Friedewald formula and direct measurement is rarely employed outside specialist centres and research projects (LDL-cholesterol was measured directly in the Heart Protection Study).

3.5 What abnormalities of lipids are seen?

The results of lipid testing are often erroneously seen as diagnoses in themselves (e.g. hypercholesterolaemia or hypertriglyceridaemia) and this probably stems from the first classification of lipid disorders proposed by Frederickson and adopted by the World Health Organization (WHO) in 1970.[4] The classification was based on observations of sera, and the levels and electrophoretic mobility of lipoprotein particles. This classification enabled much progress to be made in understanding lipoprotein metabolism; however, it was difficult to apply to the clinical setting and many grappled with its complexities.

The most useful classification of lipid disorders is into primary and secondary dyslipidaemias. The term dyslipidaemia is preferable to hyperlipidaemia because qualitative as well as quantitative abnormalities occur and, in the case of HDL-cholesterol, the abnormality is often one of low, not raised, concentration. Recently, Durrington summarised the dyslipidaemias found on lipid testing, adopting a clinical approach and grouping the disorders according to whether the biochemical pattern (phenotype) observed is mainly hypercholesterolaemia, a combined increase in cholesterol and triglycerides, mainly hypertriglyceridaemia, hypolipidaemia or secondary dyslipidaemia.[5] A full description of the primary and secondary dyslipidaemias is found in Chapter 4 but Durrington's classification of primary dyslipidaemias is shown in *Table 3.1*.

3.6 How accurate are the measurements?

A number of biological influences mean that cholesterol levels vary from day to day, week to week and year to year. In a cohort of 14 600 people with repeat cholesterol measurements, the within-person coefficient of variation after 1 year was 7.4%. This means that for an individual with a mean total cholesterol value of 6.5 mmol/L, fluctuations of up to 0.5 mmol/L either way could be found on retesting. If several readings are taken (just like repeat blood pressure testing in the diagnosis of hypertension), the effect of within-person variation is much reduced. Triglyceride levels are subject to even wider natural variation, particularly with their close temporal relationship to food intake.

In women, lipid levels vary with the menstrual cycle (both cholesterol and triglycerides tending to peak mid-cycle) and in pregnancy. Lipid concentrations also vary with the seasons, being highest in the winter and lowest in the summer (probably reflecting seasonal differences in diet and body weight). Both major and minor illnesses (including trauma and surgery) usually reduce cholesterol and raise triglycerides. The effect can be profound and rapid and, after serious illness, recovery can be delayed for as long as 3 months. For this reason the lipid levels of patients admitted with myocardial infarction (MI) are usually estimated within 24 hours to reflect pre-event status. Arguably, this is less important now as all MI victims benefit from a statin irrespective of their baseline lipid levels.

TABLE 3.1 Patterns of primary dyslipidaemia found on measurement of cholesterol, HDL-cholesterol and triglycerides

Dyslipidaemia	WHO phenotype	Diagnosis	Estimated prevalence in European adults (%)
Mainly hypercholesterolaemia	Type IIa: raised LDL	Monogenic hypercholesterolaemia: familial hypercholesterolaemia familial defective apo-B Polygenic hypercholesterolaemia	0.2 0.2 20–80
Combined hypercholesterolaemia and hypertriglyceridaemia: TG 2–10 mmol/L	Type IIb: raised VLDL and LDL	Familial combined if relatives have same pattern, otherwise simply combined hyperlipidaemia	10+
TG 5–20 mmol/L (cholesterol typically 7–12 mmol/L) TG >10 mmol/L	Type III: raised chylomicron remnants and IDL Type V: raised chylomicrons and VLDL; or type I: raised chylomicrons	Type III or remnant particle disease	0.02
Raised triglycerides alone	Type IV	Lipoprotein lipase deficiency Familial or sporadic hypertriglyceridaemia	0.1 1
Hypoalphalipoproteinaemia	None: low HDL	Often undiagnosed and associated with low HDL	10–25
Hypobetalipoproteinaemia	None: low LDL and frequently VLDL	Familial, e.g. truncated apo-B	0.01–0.1

HDL, high density lipoprotein; IDL, intermediate density lipoprotein (VLDL remnants); LDL, low density lipoprotein; TG, triglycerides; VLDL, very low density lipoprotein. After Durrington,[5] with permission from Elsevier.

As if biological variation were not enough, the situation is further complicated by analytical variation. Most laboratories operate at a coefficient of variation of about 2%.

> Taken together, both biological and analytical variation emphasise the need for repeated testing and care, particularly when decisions are being made concerning the initiation and monitoring of treatment.

3.7 How do lipid levels change according to age and gender?

Studies within populations, such as Framingham, establish that there are not only slight gender differences in lipid patterns but also more significant trends with the passage of time. American studies show total cholesterol levels in cord blood around 1.7 mmol/L, equally distributed between LDL- and HDL-cholesterol. The first 6 months of life see a rapid rise in cholesterol to about 4 mmol/L until puberty when there is a rise in LDL-cholesterol and triglycerides in both sexes and a fall in HDL-cholesterol in boys but not in girls. During adult life lipid levels continue to rise in both sexes, being higher in men until about 55 years of age when levels in women become higher. HDL-cholesterol levels remain higher at all times in women, even after the menopause. Triglycerides are higher in men until about 65 years when they become similar in both sexes.[6] These changes are summarised in *Figure 3.1.*

3.8 How often should lipid tests be repeated?

Five years probably represents a reasonable frequency for cholesterol testing for primary prevention risk assessment from age 20 to 80 years, according to overall risk. Borderline cases can vary from 1 to 5 years. For patients already on treatment with diet, testing initially every 3 months, then every 6–12 months would be reasonable. For patients on medication, testing every 4–8 weeks until target achievement, then every 12 months, would be reasonable.

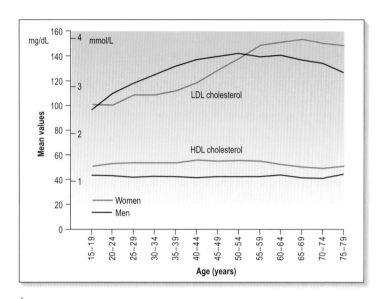

▲

Fig. 3.1 Trends in lipoprotein levels in men and women according to age. Cholesterol and LDL are significantly lower in children and results in children are likely to become higher post-puberty. (Adapted from Kannel,[6] with permission from the International Life Sciences Institute.)

PATIENT QUESTIONS

3.9 What is 'the lipid profile'?

'The lipid profile' refers to the levels of cholesterol, LDL-cholesterol, HDL-cholesterol and triglycerides measured in your blood sample. In the steady state, the absorption of cholesterol from the diet and its manufacture in the liver are precisely balanced by excretion in the faeces and, despite popular concerns, levels of both total and HDL-cholesterol are little affected by recent food consumption.

In contrast, the level of triglycerides is affected by recent food intake and remains elevated for several hours after eating fat. In healthy subjects, triglycerides will usually return to a steady level by about 6 hours and, in most individuals, by 12 hours. This is the reason why the lipid profile is usually measured after a 12-hour fast, allowing only water to offset thirst. Fasting ensures a reproducible measure in the laboratory but some commentators have argued that as human beings are hardly ever in the fasting state, fasting levels of triglycerides do not reflect the effect of a day's

PATIENT QUESTIONS

exposure. A parallel is seen in blood pressure measurement where health professionals take readings in the resting state rather than peak readings under the stresses of exertion or emotion.

3.10 How would I know if my lipid profile was abnormal?

Individuals with abnormal lipids are impossible to identify without a test. Even external signs of abnormal lipids, such as the corneal arcus and xanthelasmata (described in *Ch. 4*), are not always specific.

The interpretation of the significance of the results of a fasting lipid profile is now a skill requirement for all healthcare professionals interested in cardiovascular disease prevention. Someone with this skill will always evaluate lipid levels within the context of overall ('global') cardiovascular risk assessment. This means taking the pattern of your lipid profile into account with any other risk factors (*see Qs 2.1, 2.7 and 2.20, and Ch. 5*) to estimate your future risk of a cardiovascular event, such as a heart attack.

3.11 What levels are desirable?

There is some variation in what experts agree as desirable lipid levels but a useful guide is found in the Third Report of the Adult Treatment Panel of the National Cholesterol Education Program (NCEP ATP III) in the USA:

- 'Desirable' cholesterol is   <5.2 mmol/L (<200 mg/dL)*
- 'High' HDL-cholesterol is   >1.5 mmol/L (>60 mg/dL)
- 'Optimal' LDL-cholesterol is   <2.6 mmol/L (<100 mg/dL)*
- 'Normal' triglycerides are   <1.7 mmol/L (<150 mg/dL)

For individuals whose cardiovascular risk is such that they need lipid-lowering drugs, specific targets (goals of therapy) are set and these are reviewed in *Question 9.5.*

Many experts now believe that there should be less reliance on target achievement and more focus on delivering an absolute reduction in the cholesterol level of any individual whose level of cardiovascular risk is sufficiently high to require treatment. The positive outcome of the Heart Protection Study was based on the hypothesis that lowering LDL-cholesterol (in the end by about 1.0 mmol/L) in high-risk individuals, irrespective of their baseline levels, would effect a reduction in subsequent cardiovascular events. Similar effects are seen in the ASCOT and CARDS trials where benefits of cholesterol lowering are seen irrespective of baseline levels.

---

*UK figures were <5.0 and <3.0 mmol/L, and are now <4.0 and <2.0 mmol/L, respectively.

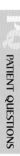

Lipid disorders

4

4.1	What are primary and secondary hyperlipidaemias?	48
4.2	What conditions cause secondary hyperlipidaemia?	50
4.3	What is the metabolic syndrome?	51
4.4	What drugs cause secondary hyperlipidaemia?	51
4.5	What is common polygenic hypercholesterolaemia (hyperlipidaemia)?	52
4.6	What are the features of familial hypercholesterolaemia?	52
4.7	How is familial hypercholesterolaemia diagnosed?	53
4.8	How can more cases of familial hypercholesterolaemia be detected?	55
4.9	What is familial defective apolipoprotein-B?	56
4.10	What are the features of familial combined hyperlipidaemia?	56
4.11	What are the features of remnant particle disease?	56
4.12	What are the features of isolated hypertriglyceridaemia?	58
4.13	What is the role of the specialist lipidologist?	60

PATIENT QUESTIONS

4.14	At what age is cardiovascular disease considered premature?	61
4.15	How are the risks of passing on genetic hyperlipidaemia defined?	61
4.16	At what age should children be screened for genetic hyperlipidaemia where there is a known family history?	63
4.17	Does identifying a genetic hyperlipidaemia make any difference?	64

4.1 What are primary and secondary hyperlipidaemias?

Various classifications of lipid disorders are possible. *Box 4.1* classifies these on the basis of the clinical (phenotypic) picture, related to elevated cholesterol or triglycerides or both, or low lipid levels.

Within these categories the dyslipidaemia may be due to a primary disturbance in lipid metabolism. However, the same patterns may be due to, or have substantial contribution from, (and therefore be secondary to) disorders such as hypothyroidism or diabetes, or from exogenous causes such as drug treatments or alcohol use. Where hypothyroidism or type 1 diabetes gives rise to dyslipidaemia this is secondary to hormone lack and can be corrected by replacement therapy. Perhaps the situation is less clear with type 2 diabetes where replacement therapy often does not correct the situation, the dyslipidaemia being part of the underlying disorder.

Secondary causes are many, but the commoner or more classical ones are given in *Box 4.2*.

BOX 4.1 Classification of dyslipidaemias

Hypercholesterolaemia

1. High LDL:
   a. Primary:
      i. Familial hypercholesterolaemia (*see* Q 4.6) – LDL receptor mutation or defective apolipoprotein B
      ii. Polygenic hypercholesterolaemia – not genetically characterised
   b. Secondary:
      i. Drug treatments
      ii. Disease states:
         — endocrine
         — renal
         — hepatic
2. High HDL:
   a. Familial
   b. Gender – moderately higher in women than in men
   c. CETP deficiency

Hypertriglyceridaemia

1. Primary:
   a. Familial hypertriglyceridaemia
2. Secondary:
   a. Physiological – pregnancy
   b. Alcohol, drugs

BOX 4.1 Classification of dyslipidaemias—cont'd

Mixed hyperlipidaemia

1. Familial
   a. Familial combined hyperlipidaemia
   b. Familial dysbetalipoproteinaemia (remnant lipaemia; type III hyperlipidaemia)
2. Secondary
   a. Insulin resistance syndrome – metabolic syndrome (*see Q 4.3 and Box 1.1*)
   b. Type 2 diabetes
   c. Drug treatments (HDL variable)
   d. Disease states
   e. Alcohol (often with higher HDL levels)

Low lipid – lipoprotein levels

1. Familial low HDL
   a. Tangier disease
   b. LCAT deficiency
   c. Apolipoprotein A deficiency
   d. Polygenic – (common)
2. Low LDL
   a. Hypobetalipoproteinaemia and abetalipoproteinaemia

CETP, cholesterol ester transfer protein; LCAT, lecithin cholesterol acyl transferase.

Primary (familial) hyperlipidaemias used to be classified by the Fredrickson taxonomy into types I, II (types IIa and IIb), III, IV and V:

- In types I and V there is very severe hypertriglyceridaemia, rare as a primary inherited defect but rather more common due to secondary causes. As a primary disorder type I is a rare condition due to lipoprotein lipase (or more rarely apolipoprotein-CII) deficiency. This leads to chylomicrons accumulating in the blood, present from childhood, and with a high risk of acute pancreatitis. In adults very low density lipoproteins (VLDLs) also accumulate (type V).
- Type II is hypercholesterolaemia when triglycerides are normal (type IIa) or modestly elevated (type IIb). The inherited form is familial hypercholesterolaemia.
- Type III lipaemia is a rare condition where both cholesterol and triglycerides are elevated, often each elevated in the 6–10 mmol/L range. About 1 in 100 of the population has inherited one copy of a particular form of apolipoprotein E (apo-E2) from each parent. Those

people homozygous for apo-E2 have rather slower clearance by the liver from the blood of VLDL remnants. About 2% of these people (and therefore about 1 in 5000 of the population) fail to clear remnants that accumulate with severe mixed lipaemia.

■ In type IV hyperlipidaemia there are moderate elevations of both cholesterol and triglycerides, due to elevation of triglyceride-rich lipoproteins (VLDLs and intermediate density lipoproteins, IDLs) and LDL. This can be an inherited trait. Much more commonly it has substantial secondary contributors (e.g. obesity, diabetes, alcohol excess, untreated hypothyroidism) and may be seen often in metabolic syndrome patients (*see Q 4.3 and Box 1.1*).

4.2 What conditions cause secondary hyperlipidaemia?

Hyperlipidaemia may be due to an inherited predisposition, either single gene (monogenic) or to the interaction of multiple genes (polygenic), and is then considered to be a primary hyperlipidaemia.

Secondary hyperlipidaemias (*Box 4.2*) result from the effects of other diseases influencing the lipid profile, such as hepatic, renal or endocrine (e.g. hypothyroidism and diabetes) disease.

 Environmental, dietary and lifestyle factors may bring to light or may exacerbate either primary or secondary hyperlipidaemias. Sedentary lifestyles, poor diet, excess alcohol and obesity may all contribute here.

Some drug treatments – such as thiazides and beta-blockers, hormone treatments, steroid therapy, retinoids for dermatological conditions and

---

BOX 4.2 Secondary hyperlipidaemias and dyslipidaemias

■ Hormonal – hypothyroid
■ Steroids – Cushing's disease or syndrome (including exogenous therapy or misuse)
■ Renal disease – renal failure, nephrotic syndrome
■ Liver disease – cholestasis, alcoholic liver disease, metabolic syndrome, non-alcoholic fatty liver disease (NAFLD)
■ Obesity
■ Drug therapies:
  — oestrogen, anti-oestrogens
  — retinoic acid
  — protease inhibitors
  — thiazides
  — beta-blockers
  — ciclosporin
  — psychotropic agents (some)

retroviral treatments – may bring out hyperlipidaemias in susceptible individuals.

The most common secondary hyperlipidaemias are found with diabetes, hepatic and renal disease, and endocrine disorders such as hypothyroidism.

4.3   What is the metabolic syndrome?

The term 'metabolic syndrome' is applied to a constellation of abnormalities that include hypertension, mixed hyperlipidaemia (with raised triglycerides and low high density lipoprotein-cholesterol), glucose intolerance (and diabetes mellitus), central adiposity (variously defined), insulin resistance and premature cardiovascular disease. Other components may also be present, such as hyperuricaemia and gout, polycystic ovarian syndrome and previous gestational diabetes.

As a result of these wide-ranging abnormalities, different definitions have been applied, but perhaps the one most often used nowadays is that from the US National Cholesterol Education Program's Third Report from the Adult Treatment Panel (NCEP ATP-III)[1] (*see Box 1.1*). The reason for concern about metabolic syndrome is the constellation of conditions that accompanies it. Associated with the insulin resistance is a high risk of developing impaired glucose tolerance and diabetes. If not tackled, this risk and the other problems cause premature morbidity and mortality.

Different races may need adjustment of these definitions for an equivalent risk profile. Thus in populations from an Indian subcontinent origin, overweight and obese may be defined as a body mass index (BMI) of >23 and >27 for females and males, respectively, rather than >25 and >30 respectively for Caucasian populations. Similarly in the Japanese, equivalent values for waist circumference might be taken as >85 and >90 cm for females and males, respectively.

4.4   What drugs cause secondary hyperlipidaemia?

Many drugs can contribute to a secondary hyperlipidaemia, or can exacerbate a primary or other secondary hyperlipidaemia. The possibility of leading to or exacerbating an existing lipaemia should be considered when drug treatments are used. The major drugs groups likely to contribute are listed in *Box 4.2*.

As in pregnancy, where an hypertriglyceridaemic state is common (and physiological), use of oestrogens can cause the same problems. Similar patterns occur with ciclosporin and retinoic acid. The retroviral agents (the protease inhibitors) also cause hypertriglyceridaemia or mixed lipaemia, as do thiazide diuretics and beta-blockers. Some drugs for psychoses can also raise triglycerides (olanzapine and others in the class).

Hypercholesterolaemia or mixed lipaemias can occur with steroids, thiazides and anti-oestrogens.

4.5 What is common polygenic hypercholesterolaemia (hyperlipidaemia)?

Polygenic hypercholesterolaemia is poorly defined, and the genetic or molecular basis is not well understood. However, it is clear that perhaps half the variability in blood lipid and lipoprotein levels has a genetic contribution. While such genetic predispositions clearly run through families, environmental and lifestyle contributions can play a large part in exacerbating the dyslipidaemia.

Although such patterns of dyslipidaemia are evident in families, the phenotypic expression can vary within different family members, or indeed in an individual with time, depending on current lifestyle and other factors. While one member of the family may be found to have high cholesterol levels, in other situations (e.g. a more sedentary lifestyle, weight increase or changed diet) triglycerides may also be raised with a mixed hyperlipidaemia.

When an individual is found to have a dyslipidaemia, it is important to consider other (first degree) family members, especially where the proband or family members have or have had cardiovascular disease or suffered sudden death. With a polygenic contribution one may find some family members with elevated cholesterol, high triglycerides or a mixed lipaemia (and this may then represent familial combined hyperlipidaemia).

4.6 What are the features of familial hypercholesterolaemia?

Familial hypercholesterolaemia (FH) is due to a gene defect in the receptor for low density lipoprotein (LDL) or at times due to a (familial) defective apolipoprotein-B (*see Q 4.9*).

In the heterozygous state it is present in 1 in 500 of the population in most countries. The homozygous state then has an incidence of 1 per million, although because of reduced life expectancy its prevalence is substantially less. In some communities, either from a 'founder' effect or from intermarriage (first cousin marriages) the frequency is substantially increased. Such communities include the French Canadians, the Afrikaans and the Lebanese.

Untreated, in the heterozygote, the first cardiac (cardiovascular) event has occurred by age 50 years in 50% of males, 50% having died by age 60 years. In females, disease events occur approximately 5–10 years later. There is variability in these ages, and events in some families track at a substantially earlier age than in other families, and this needs to be assessed in considering the young age at which to begin pharmacological intervention.

The homozygote is rare, but is very severely affected. Untreated nearly all are dead by the age of 20, but aggressive drug treatment and LDL-apheresis (*see Qs 7.31 and 7.32*) can markedly extend (at least double) their life expectancy. These individuals usually develop coronary heart disease (CHD) in childhood.

4.7 How is familial hypercholesterolaemia diagnosed?

Familial hypercholesterolaemia is diagnosed by the finding of significant hypercholesterolaemia (>7.5 mmol/L) (or LDL-cholesterol >4.9 mmol/L) with one other feature. Definite FH requires either the near-pathognomonic tendon xanthomata or genetic evidence (*Box 4.3*). Probable FH requires the hypercholesterolaemia (above) together with a family history either of FH or of premature CHD.

While 1 in 500 of the population has FH, no more than 20% have been found. A proportion of FH patients will have cholesterol deposition in extensor tendons of the hands as seen in *Figure 4.1*. Often they are small and are best identified by palpation over the tendons while the fingers are passively flexed and extended when the xanthoma may be felt moving.

BOX 4.3 Diagnostic features of familial hypercholesterolaemia

1. Total cholesterol >7.5 mmol/L (treated or untreated) in an adult (child >6.7 mmol/L) or an LDL-cholesterol >4.9 mmol/L in an adult (child 4.0 mmol/L)
2. Tendon xanthoma(ta) in first or second degree relative (*see Fig. 4.1*)
3. DNA evidence of an LDL receptor mutation or of familial defective apo-B100 (FDB)
4. Family history of myocardial infarction <50 years in second degree relative or <60 years in first degree relative
5. Family history

'Definite' FH requires both (1) and (2), or (1) and (3)
'Probable' FH requires both (1) and (4), or (1) and (5)

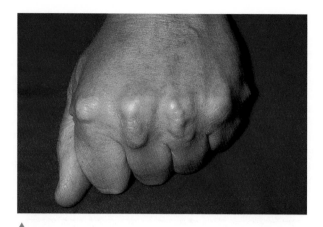

▲

Fig. 4.1 Tendon xanthomata in the extensor tendons of the hand in familial hypercholesterolaemia.

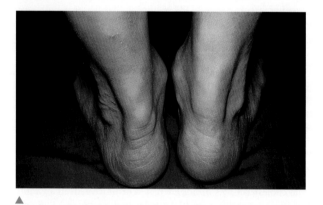

▲

Fig. 4.2 Achilles tendon xanthomata are found in some patients with familial hypercholesterolaemia, and confirm this diagnosis.

Thickening of the Achilles tendon a little above its insertion into the calcaneum (in the absence of a history of local injury) is a further tendon xanthoma site. Achilles tendons should be no thicker than the patient's little finger (*Fig. 4.2*). Tendon xanthomata are pathognomonic of FH. When FH is diagnosed family testing is mandatory, since each first degree relative has a 50:50 chance of being affected.

Lipid deposition in the eyelids is a feature of hyperlipidaemia, perhaps more commonly in type II and type IV patients, and at times with

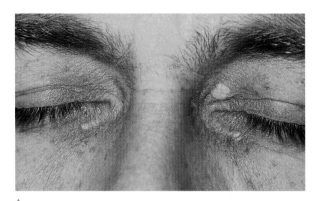

Fig. 4.3 Lipid deposit(s) – xanthelasma(ta) – (especially in younger patients) are suggestive, but not diagnostic, of a dyslipidaemia.

secondary contributing factors for the dyslipidaemia. However, a xanthelasma (xanthelasmata) may occur in individuals without significant dyslipidaemia, but abnormal lipids are quite likely in young patients with xanthelasmata (*Fig. 4.3*). A further eye sign that again is not specific but may indicate a significant dyslipidaemia is premature corneal arcus.

> People fulfilling these criteria should not have their cardiovascular risk calculated by the primary prevention charts as, untreated, they have very high risks, and should be considered as secondary prevention patients requiring treatment. Many of these patients will justify referral to a specialist clinic at least initially. They need counselling about their and their relatives' risks, and family screening is essential. They should also be referred to the cholesterol charity – HEART UK – for support (*see Appendix*).

4.8 How can more cases of familial hypercholesterolaemia be detected?

When an individual with possible FH is suspected, a formal assessment for this possible condition should be undertaken (*see Box 4.3*). Such FH individuals and their families require screening by their medical advisors, potential referral to their local specialist centre and effective screening of their first degree relatives (and in turn of the relatives of any affected such first degree relatives). The medical practitioner responsible for the proband's care has an ethical duty to check that the proband has passed on the information to the relatives concerned, who will often be under the care of different medical teams.

In 2004 the UK government (through the Department of Health) set up a pilot study in several parts of the country to investigate the best way to arrange such cascade screening (*see* Q 2.16), but clinicians should continue to undertake this role in the meantime.

4.9 What is familial defective apolipoprotein-B?

While most patients who present with the clinical picture of FH have a defect in the gene for the LDL receptor (currently more than 700 defects have been identified), such defects have not been identified in some individuals or families.

However, in some families the LDL receptor is normal, and abnormal LDL protein has been found. These patients have an abnormal LDL apolipoprotein-B which does not bind to the LDL receptor which is normal. The clinical result is the same, for the circulating LDL cannot be removed efficaciously, and the clinical picture of FH with high circulating cholesterol and LDL-cholesterol results in premature cardiovascular disease.

4.10 What are the features of familial combined hyperlipidaemia?

There are no diagnostic clinical features of familial combined hyperlipidaemia. These patients do not have the near-diagnostic tendon xanthomata of familial hypercholesterolaemia. They may have premature corneal arcus or xanthelasmata, but these are not diagnostic, and their absence also does not help.

In these individuals elevated cholesterol and also triglycerides are found, with a significantly increased risk of vascular disease. The triglycerides are usually moderately rather than severely raised. Often there is a family history of premature vascular disease and/or hyperlipidaemia. The pattern of raised cholesterol, raised triglycerides, or both raised, may vary within an individual over time, partly reflecting changes in diet, lifestyle, weight, exercise or alcohol. The hyperlipidaemia also varies in different members of the proband's family.

4.11 What are the features of remnant particle disease?

Remnant particles are the lipoproteins that are formed as the triglyceride-rich lipoproteins – chylomicrons and very low density lipoproteins (VLDL) – are catabolised. These remnant particles normally are removed quickly from the circulation, but in remnant lipaemia they accumulate in the blood, often being termed intermediate density lipoproteins (IDL). They are particularly atherogenic, substantially increasing the risk for CHD and peripheral vascular disease.

The condition of remnant particle disease (or remnant hyperlipidaemia) has also been termed type III hyperlipidaemia or familial dysbetalipoproteinaemia (there being an inherited predisposition).

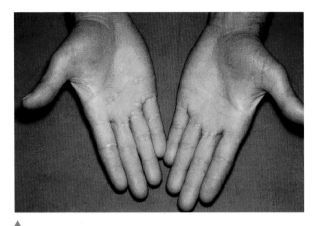

Fig. 4.4 Palmar crease xanthomata in type III hyperlipidaemia (remnant hyperlipidaemia; familial dysbetalipoproteinaemia).

Clinically these individuals have substantial elevation in both cholesterol and triglyceride, these often being in the 7–10 mmol/L range, although they will be outside these values on occasions. Sometimes there may be xanthelasmata and premature corneal arcus, although the presence or absence of these does not make or break the diagnosis. However, when the dyslipidaemia is more severe some individuals do develop classical and diagnostic xanthomata (*Fig 4.4*). Such palmar skin crease xanthomata are diagnostic, but are often not present and can be quite subtle. Palmar xanthomata are classically in the skin creases of the palm and in the flexor creases at the metacarpophalangeal and interphalangeal joints, and have a golden yellow colour. This colour is quite subtle, but is best seen, photographing less well. When more severe, there may also be the more raised yellowy-white xanthomata as seen in *Figure 4.4*. These are non-painful. They resolve quite quickly with treatment, and good quality, lower fat, calorie-reduced, weight-reducing diets are often sufficient. In resistant cases, after exclusion (or treatment) of other contributory secondary causes, then a fibrate is the treatment of choice, statins being a reserve option.

The genetic background to remnant lipaemia is an inheritance of an abnormality in the apolipoprotein-E (apo-E) gene. Apo-E exists in a number of isoforms, of which the commonest is apo-E3. One single amino acid substitution in apo-E gives an isoform, apo-E2, which is less well recognised by the liver apo-E receptor. Lipoproteins with apo-E2 are then more slowly removed. About 1% of the population is homozygous, having two copies of apo-E2. In about 1–2% of these individuals the removal of remnant particles is sufficiently delayed for severe accumulation to occur in the plasma (with the resultant clinical and pathological features). While it is not entirely clear why only a few individuals with this inherited pattern develop the clinical pathological condition, there is almost always some other inherited or secondary dyslipidaemia, or there is obesity, alcohol excess, diabetes, hypothyroidism, etc. that further stresses the lipid clearance mechanisms.

Treatment of these individuals is essential, with correction of any secondary causes. Dietary management may suffice, but the drug of choice here is a fibrate (such as fenofibrate) although a statin can be helpful second line in some (*see Ch. 7*). Siblings should be checked as they also may have the condition.

4.12 What are the features of isolated hypertriglyceridaemia?

Isolated hypertriglyceridaemia is often silent, and may not have clinical features or disease. It may be familial. Other disorders or lifestyle issues may exacerbate it. In the severe form, when triglycerides rise above 10 mmol/L and especially above 20 mmol/L, the risk of acute pancreatitis is greatly increased. Once an attack of pancreatitis has occurred, such individuals are much more prone to recurrent attacks. It is unclear why some individuals with such severe hypertriglyceridaemia have acute pancreatitis and others do not. When an individual is admitted with acute pancreatitis the possibility of severe hypertriglyceridaemia must be considered. The laboratory should report 'lipaemic serum', but if not measured promptly the triglycerides may settle quite quickly with an acutely ill patient receiving just intravenous fluids. Alcohol may be a feature in the genesis of the hypertriglyceridaemia and in the acute pancreatitis itself in some individuals.

Patients with severe insulin resistance commonly have severe and central obesity. This can be associated with hypertension, lipid abnormalities (usually a mixed lipaemia with raised triglycerides and low HDL), abnormal glucose tolerance, hyperuricaemia and gout, and premature vascular disease. Some of these individuals manifest this insulin resistance with acanthosis nigricans, and in these patients it is *not* indicative of occult malignancy. The skin becomes thickened, velvety and brownish-yellow discoloured in axillae (*Fig. 4.5*) and inguinal areas, and over the back of the neck.

With severely elevated triglycerides (10–20 mmol/L and above) individuals may get eruptive skin xanthomata, though they are not usually as extensive as seen in *Figure 4.6*. These are painless pinkish macular–papular spots which can appear over a few days, and with calorie restriction can fade and resolve over a similar time as triglycerides fall to single figures (mmol/L). They are normally not symptomatic.

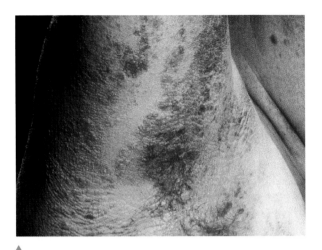

Fig. 4.5 Acanthosis nigricans, a velvety brownish-yellow thickening of the skin in axillae, inguinal areas and back of the neck, can be seen in very obese and severely insulin-resistant patients, when it is *not* indicative of occult malignancy.

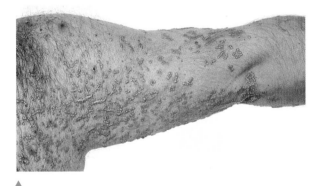

Fig. 4.6 Eruptive xanthomata occur in some patients with severe (type I or type V) hypertriglyceridaemia (>20 mmol/L).

Atrophy of adipose tissue may be a rare acquired abnormality in some people. Various forms are recognised, which may be subtotal or total, and may for example spare the face. Some individuals have pseudohypertrophy of muscle. Almost all these individuals develop severe insulin resistance and may often eventually develop glucose intolerance and diabetes. Severe hypertriglyceridaemia is often found. While not licensed for this indication, the thiazolidinediones can be very helpful in improving the metabolic picture, although a substantial increase in adipose tissue may then occur. In this circumstance, these drugs should be initiated by specialist clinics.

Severe isolated hypertriglyceridaemia is not normally associated with premature macrovascular disease, and the triglyceride may be associated with only moderate increases in cholesterol. As all lipoproteins will contain both cholesterol and triglycerides in varying amounts, when the triglyceride-rich lipoproteins are markedly raised the cholesterol is also pulled up somewhat (by roughly 1 mmol/L for every 5 mmol/L increase in triglycerides).

Treatment is calorie restriction, attendance to lifestyle and exercise and reduction or removal of alcohol once secondary precipitating causes have been excluded. Fibrates, fish oils and nicotinic acid have pharmaceutical roles in some patients.

Rarely (about 1 in 1 000 000) there may be an inherited abnormality or absence of the main plasma enzyme responsible for the clearance of triglycerides from circulating triglyceride-rich lipoproteins, called lipoprotein lipase (LPL). Rarer still, with an identical picture and with consequences as in LPL deficiency, is a deficiency of apolipoprotein-CII which is an activator of LPL. These individuals may only show accumulation of chylomicrons, but in older age and with increasing obesity and similar environmental changes may also accumulate VLDLs. Treatment here is very severe restriction of fat in the diet down to less than 10% of calories. This is quite demanding, bearing in mind that the usual 'low fat' diet recommended for hyperlipidaemia restricts fat to <30% of calories. Such patients need substantial dietary input, and should be under the care of a specialist lipid clinic.

4.13 What is the role of the specialist lipidologist?

In most teaching and district general hospitals there will now be a lipid service, which may be run from endocrine, cardiac and gastroenterology departments and/or with the clinical biochemistry department. This clinic is more likely to provide a macrovascular prevention service addressing all the risk factors, rather than just the lipid abnormalities.

In a smaller number of centres there will also be a specialist lipidologist providing expertise in the investigation of the rarer dyslipidaemias and in the management of the patient with difficult lipid problems. The lipidologist may be a consultant physician or a consultant clinical biochemist, and there may be a jointly provided service. Clinical research will often be undertaken, and in some units laboratory-based research also.

Patients with inherited dyslipidaemias and their families are likely to benefit from a specialist referral, the confirmation of the specific disorder, the initiation and stabilisation of treatment, and sometimes longer term shared follow-up with the primary care team. Inherited dyslipidaemias also give rise to the need for counselling about inherited risks, and about the age at which screening and treatment should be considered in children and young adults. Additionally, complicated patients with poorly responding dyslipidaemias, those with apparent treatment side effects, and those with multiple medications are likely to attend. With some secondary dyslipidaemias, the specialist lipidologist will be able to provide management advice.

With some patients the decision as to the likelihood of treatment benefit, or of cost-benefit, together with a patient's own concerns about lifelong treatment, can be facilitated by a specialist consultation. There are many individuals at moderate risk where pharmacotherapy treatment decisions may be finely balanced and substantially influenced by patient choice.

PATIENT QUESTIONS

4.14   At what age is cardiovascular disease considered premature?

For many people an avoidable illness can be considered premature. When considering the criteria for the diagnosis of familial hypercholesterolaemia (FH), a family history of a myocardial infarction at less than 50 years in a second degree relative or at less than 60 years in first degree relative is used with an elevated cholesterol to make the diagnosis of probable FH.

However, in other situations (such as when using the Joint British Societies' charts for the calculation of risk for primary prevention of coronary heart disease) premature vascular disease is defined as before the age of 55 years in the male and 65 years in the female. If a first degree relative has such a premature history then the proband whose risk has been estimated from the charts should have that risk augmented by at least 50%.

As the average life expectancy of the population has been increasing steadily over the last 20–30 years by about 2–3 months every year, perhaps the age at which cardiovascular disease is considered premature should also be extended. Premature disease could be considered to have occurred when a previously fit individual has a first event, for in prevention programmes the intention is to increase the number of healthy disease-free years.

4.15   How are the risks of passing on genetic hyperlipidaemia defined?

The risks of passing on a genetic hyperlipidaemia will depend on the particular lipid disorder being considered.

Familial hypercholesterolaemia

Perhaps the most straightforward example is familial hypercholesterolaemia. A gene codes for the cell receptor that removes LDL-cholesterol (the so-called 'bad' cholesterol when present in excess). Each individual has two sets of genes, one from each parent. If one of the LDL receptor genes is defective then the person's blood cholesterol tends to double as only half the LDL receptors are operative. A person with one abnormal gene and LDL receptor (and one normal one) is said to be 'heterozygous', and this occurs in around 1 in 500 of the population. Much higher LDL levels are found when both receptors are faulty (termed 'homozygous'), but this is very rare, being about 1 in a million of the population. These patients may develop cholesterol thickening and lumps in some of the muscle tendons (*see Figs 4.1 and 4.2*)

If a person has one faulty gene and one normal gene (the heterozygote state) and has children (and assuming their other parent is normal), then any child will have a 50:50 chance of having the abnormal gene. If a person has one faulty gene, this means that one of the parents will also have had the faulty gene, and any brother or sister of that person will also have a 50:50 chance of having inherited the condition.

The reason why the homozygote state is so rare is that such a person has to have inherited two abnormal genes, one from each parent. This means that the parents are both heterozygous, a chance of 1 in 500 multiplied by 1 in 500, i.e. 1 in 250 000. Any children have a 1 in 4 chance of inheriting two normal genes (and the condition will then be passed on no further), or a 2 in 4 chance of having one abnormal gene and one normal (i.e. being a heterozygote), and a 1 in 4 chance of unfortunately having two abnormal genes (a homozygote) – this overall risk therefore being 1 in a million.

In familial hypercholesterolaemia therefore, the message is almost always that any first degree relative of an affected individual has a 50:50 chance of also being affected as in tossing a coin for heads or tails.

Remnant lipaemia

A different inheritance occurs in remnant lipaemia, and this is rarer. Here one of the proteins that controls the removal of the circulating cholesterol and blood fats is abnormal because of an altered gene, but a lipid disorder in the blood occurs only if the gene inherited from both parents is abnormal. This occurs in about 1 in 100 of the population. Normal blood cholesterol and blood fats are maintained with just one normal gene. Indeed, in nearly all individuals normal blood levels can be maintained with both genes abnormal. It seems that it requires the addition of a different defect, or a poor diet, sedentary lifestyle, excess alcohol or obesity before the abnormal protein does not 'cope' and a hyperlipidaemia results. These people may develop fatty deposits in their palms and fingers (*see Fig. 4.4*).

The chance of passing this on to children is therefore quite small, as the other parent is not likely to be affected and, even if so affected, most children will not develop abnormal lipid levels. However, if a person has the condition then it is important to examine the brothers and sisters as they do have a 25% chance of also having the disorder, and may or may not then have developed the abnormal blood levels. If brothers and sisters are normal, and the apolipoprotein E isoforms have not been measured, then the siblings need to have lipid re-measurement every few years (e.g. 2–5 years).

Polygenic lipaemia (fats raised due to small effects of many genes)

More difficult is the most common situation about inheritance. In most people abnormal blood fat and cholesterol levels result from a complex inheritance with small contributions from many genes, and how these make their contributions is not understood. In these situations the environment and lifestyle of the family members may influence whether they develop abnormal blood lipid levels, for example by being overweight, inactive, eating poorly or taking excess alcohol. Where family members are found to have higher levels of blood lipids, then other members of the family should have theirs checked, but also should do their best to follow a healthy lifestyle.

4.16 At what age should children be screened for genetic hyperlipidaemia where there is a known family history?

Most hyperlipidaemias do not manifest clinically until adulthood, often not until the third or fourth decade or later. For most individuals screening in childhood is neither appropriate nor useful.

The one exception, and a very important one, is in the inherited condition called *familial hypercholesterolaemia* (FH). This condition affects 1 in 500 of the population, and the abnormal doubling of the cholesterol level is present from birth. FH results in early heart and vascular disease, often in the fifties. This age does vary quite considerably in different families, and clearly if considerable heart disease has occurred early in a family (e.g. in their thirties), it is most important to make an early diagnosis and start treatment.

While FH can be diagnosed at birth, testing is less reliable in the first year of life, and dietary modification would rarely be undertaken before the age of 5 years. An important reason is that babies and young children need a full fat diet to get enough nourishment and calories during early growth years, and should not have any interference in their diets. Later in childhood, and if a blood sample needs to be taken for another reason it would be reasonable to measure the cholesterol. In most families where FH is recognised, testing in children tends to be done between the ages of 8 and 18 years. The blood levels tend to be lower in children before puberty, and this needs to be remembered when the value is interpreted.

The reason for testing at this age is that treatment is usually commenced in the late teens or early twenties so that there are not too many untreated adult years of life with high cholesterol levels. If the family history is more severe than average, and if heart attacks or heart disease have occurred in members of the family before the age of 40 years, then drug treatment may be recommended from the early teens, especially in boys (males tend to get the heart problems 5–10 years earlier than females). Drug treatment with non-absorbed resins (colestyramine and colestipol) can be started earlier in childhood, but these are not that easy to take and can upset the stomach. The new drug, ezetimibe, is licensed for children aged over 10 years (*see* Qs 7.21–7.23). Current treatment therefore is with statins that partly block the production of cholesterol in the body. When statins are given to young women they should be advised to stop the drug from the time of conception planning to the end of breast feeding, to avoid any moderate risk to the foetus/baby (*see* Q 7.5). Management of these high risk adolescents and children, and their families, should be undertaken by specialists in the area.

4.17 Does identifying a genetic hyperlipidaemia make any difference?

Identifying an inherited hyperlipidaemia (i.e. high levels of cholesterol or fats in the blood) does have benefits. For example in one of the inherited conditions, *familial hypercholesterolaemia*, the elevated cholesterol does not develop in adulthood but has been present from birth. As a result this condition leads to particularly premature heart disease, and early diagnosis and early treatment have substantial benefits for the individual.

Understanding that there is a particular genetic disorder may also guide treatments. For example, *remnant hyperlipidaemia* will often respond well to diet and lifestyle changes but when not fully successful the condition is normally best treated with a fibrate drug rather than a statin.

Another important reason for identifying an inherited disorder is to ensure that family members who may be affected are screened. Even when it is uncertain whether a person's hyperlipidaemia is inherited or not, it is important that parents, brothers and sisters, and children (at least adult offspring) have a fasting lipid profile measured. The doctor or nurse will ask someone with a high blood lipid level to tell their relatives and persuade them to have the test done. It is important also for these blood test results in family members to be discussed with their own doctors. In hospital specialist clinics a patient will often be asked to bring back to the clinic the values in their relatives to help identify if there is an inherited pattern. Indeed, in the UK a cascade screening project to identify family members with familial hypercholesterolaemia was started in 2004 under the auspices of the Department of Health.

Identifying individuals for treatment

5.1	What is the difference between absolute and relative risk?	66
5.2	What is global cardiovascular risk assessment?	66
5.3	How is an individual's absolute risk of cardiovascular disease assessed?	66
5.4	How accurate is cardiovascular risk assessment?	67
5.5	How can the accuracy of risk assessment be improved?	72
5.6	At what threshold should treatment be initiated?	73
5.7	Can ethnicity be quantified?	74

PATIENT QUESTIONS

5.8	How can I get my cardiovascular risk assessed?	75
5.9	What is 'primary prevention'?	75
5.10	What is 'secondary prevention'?	76
5.11	What factors determine the level at which intervention is offered?	76

5.1 What is the difference between absolute and relative risk?

Absolute risk is defined as the probability that an individual will experience an event during a specified period. Relative risk is the number of times an event is more or less likely to occur in one group, compared to another. For example, the absolute chance of winning the lottery is very low but the relative chance is doubled by buying a second ticket. However, because millions of tickets are purchased, the absolute chance of winning remains very low. In clinical terms, an intervention may halve the incidence of a disease, but if the disease is rare the intervention would need to be offered to many people for only a small number to benefit. Despite the dramatic relative risk reduction, the intervention may not be justified.

5.2 What is global cardiovascular risk assessment?

It is only recently that recommendations for preventing vascular disease have switched focus from the identification and management of individual risk factors (particularly high blood pressure and cholesterol) to the assessment and management of absolute cardiovascular risk. This takes into account the complex and synergistic relationship between risk factors and their combined or global contribution to the likelihood of a cardiovascular event.

Global absolute cardiovascular risk assessment is able to derive a prediction of the absolute cardiovascular risk of an individual over a period of time (usually 10 years) by mathematically relating the levels of their contributory risk factors to the known outcomes of similar profiles observed in large cohort studies. Assessing cardiovascular risk is not intuitive and by implementing a systematic approach based on absolute risk, health professionals can prioritise treatment to those who will benefit most. For example, the absolute 10-year cardiovascular risk of a male smoker, 65 years old, with a blood pressure of 176/96 mmHg, a cholesterol of 6.2 mmol/L and high density lipoprotein (HDL) cholesterol of 1.2 mmol/L, is 50.8%. In contrast, the risk of a 38-year-old female smoker with a blood pressure of 170/102 mmHg and the same lipid values is only 7.7%.

5.3 How is an individual's absolute risk of cardiovascular disease assessed?

Much of our understanding of the multifactorial aetiology of cardiovascular disease comes from observations from the Framingham cohort of ultimately over 10 000 men and women whose continuing screening has contributed much to the determination of the net and joint effects of cardiovascular risk factors. The data were used to derive mathematical equations from which printed charts, point scores or computer programs were evolved as support tools for health professionals assessing cardiovascular risk.

In contrast to the British[1] and American[2] risk assessment methods, which are based on the Framingham function, new European guidelines[3] use the SCORE (Systematic Coronary Risk Evaluation) system.[4] SCORE is derived from the datasets of 12 large prospective European cohort studies of over 250 000 individuals with more than 7000 fatal cardiovascular events. Two versions are available, one for low-risk countries (Belgium, France, Greece, Italy, Luxembourg, Spain, Switzerland and Portugal) and one for the remaining, higher-risk countries. Examples of the Joint British Societies' and the European charts are shown in *Figures 5.1* and *5.2*.

All three systems are used to calculate absolute risk for the *primary* prevention of cardiovascular disease only. Those with pre-existing vascular disease should be offered automatic secondary prevention interventions and all three guidelines recognise diabetes as a coronary heart disease (CHD) equivalent. The risk factors integrated in each assessment system are shown in *Table 5.1*.

The guidelines all recognise that cardiovascular risk may be higher than indicated in the chart:

- as the individual approaches the next age category
- where there is evidence of atherosclerosis in asymptomatic individuals (e.g. CT scan, ultrasound)
- in subjects with a strong family history of vascular disease
- in subjects with low HDL-cholesterol, raised triglycerides, impaired glucose tolerance and with raised levels of fibrinogen, C-reactive protein (CRP), homocysteine, apolipoprotein B or lipoprotein(a)
- in obese and sedentary subjects.

5.4   How accurate is cardiovascular risk assessment?

Despite being derived from a North American population, the Framingham function has mostly been associated with a reasonable prediction of risk in northern European countries, including the UK, and has been shown to correctly identify 85% of people who develop CHD with a 30% false positive rate.[5]

However, when applied to the database of 6643 healthy men, aged 40–59 years, in the British Regional Heart Study, the correlation between predicted risk and subsequent CHD events is poor.[6] The Framingham equations overpredict fatal and non-fatal CHD events by 47% and 57% respectively and the authors suggest that a correction factor reflecting the overestimation should be applied to calculations for the UK population.

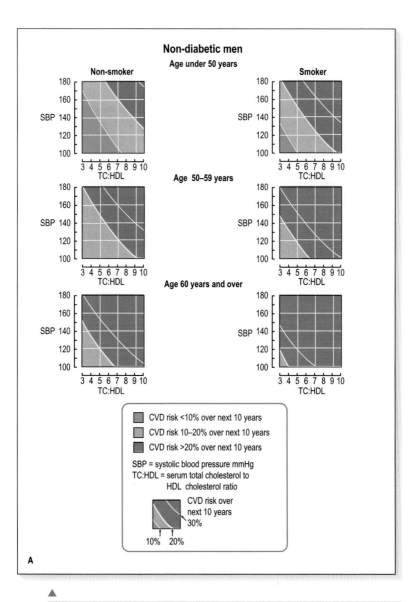

Fig. 5.1 Joint British Societies' cardiovascular disease (CVD) risk prediction charts: A, in non-diabetic men.

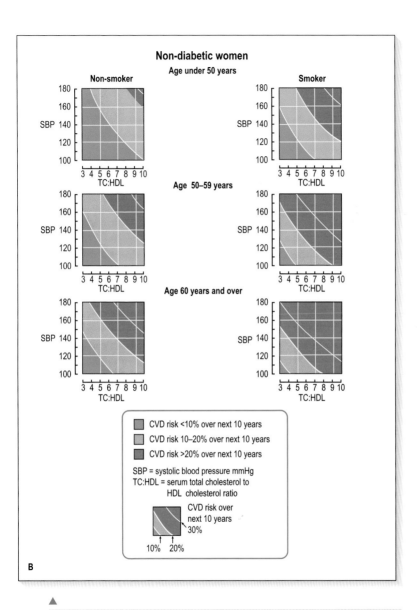

Fig. 5.1, cont'd Joint British Societies' cardiovascular disease (CVD) risk prediction charts: **B**, in non-diabetic women. SBP, systolic blood pressure mmHg; TC:HDL, serum total cholesterol to HDL-cholesterol ratio. (From the University of Manchester Department of Medical Illustration, with permission.)

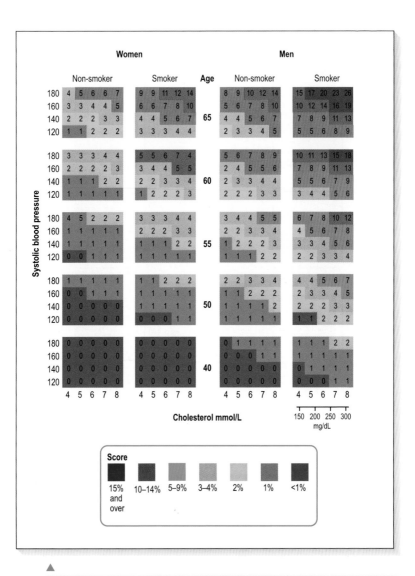

Fig. 5.2 10-year risk of fatal cardiovascular disease: populations at low cardiovascular disease risk (chart based on total cholesterol). (From Conroy et al.[4] with permission from the European Society of Cardiology.)

TABLE 5.1 Inclusion of risk factors and type of risk assessed in major risk assessment systems

Risk factor	Joint British Societies	NCEP ATP III (point score)	European Society of Cardiology
Age	Yes	Yes	Yes
Gender	Yes	Yes	Yes
Smoking	Yes	Yes	Yes
Systolic blood pressure	Yes	Yes	Yes
Total cholesterol	No	Yes	Yes
HDL-cholesterol	No	Yes	No
Cholesterol/HDL-cholesterol ratio	Yes	No	Yes (option)
Risk assessed	10-year CV risk	10-year CHD risk	10-year CV death

CHD, coronary heart disease; CV, cardiovascular; HDL, high density lipoprotein; NCEP ATP III, National Cholesterol Education Program (Adult Treatment Panel III).

The main reason why there is a difference between predicted and actual outcomes is probably historic. Framingham data were collected between 1968 and 1975 and since then actual CHD mortality has fallen, probably partly as a result of the institution of increasing numbers of preventative interventions. The differences, however, must modify the illusion of precision that some health professionals attribute to the calculations and should allow clinicians to add their clinical judgement when assessing individual cases.

Other criticisms largely stem from the limitations imposed by the study of a single population and its translation for use in others. Critics have pointed out that the Framingham function:

- is less accurate in low-risk populations
- is more accurate in older rather than younger subjects
- underestimates risk in ethnic groups
- is unreliable where extremes of risk factors are present (e.g. BP >180/110 mmHg or the high lipid levels of the familial dyslipidaemias); new Joint British Societies' guidelines[1] suggest automatic treatment when systolic blood pressure is >160 mmHg or the total cholesterol:HDL-cholesterol ratio is >7
- treats smoking as a dichotomous variable and does not account for the dose-dependent effect of smoking or the position of a lifelong smoker who has just stopped

■ does not account for the effects of an adverse family history, obesity or a sedentary lifestyle.

The SCORE system (*see Q 5.3*) also includes several of the same limitations and adds the methodological difficulties of extrapolating from a number of heterogeneous constituent population studies. In addition, health professionals are concerned with preventing morbidity and preserving quality of life as well as preventing death and it remains to be seen, in Europe, whether SCORE (which focuses only on cardiovascular death) or Framingham-based systems become adopted.

5.5 How can the accuracy of risk assessment be improved?

The risk assessment tools described here are all designed to calculate the absolute risk of CHD or cardiovascular disease over 10 years. As absolute risk increases with age, age becomes the dominant risk predictor in 10-year assessment and therefore selection for treatment. This ignores the fact that atherosclerosis is a lifelong disease and the risk factor profile which causes it may be present from an early age, albeit at lower levels of absolute risk. For younger patients, new Joint British Societies' recommendations suggest extrapolating current risk factors to age 49 and the European guidelines to age 60. Mathematical models, using lifetime risk calculations, can be used to predict the age at which starting treatment for an individual will provide maximum benefit, but these are in their infancy.

Given the geographical variation in cardiovascular disease, both between and even within countries, risk predictors are only as good as the populations on which they are based and the shortcomings of the Framingham database have been discussed (*see Q 5.4*). Risk predictors that take into account local data are ideal but represent an enormous organisational undertaking.

BOX 5.1 Major risk factors for coronary heart disease

Risk factor	Population attributable risk (%)
Apo-B/apo-AI ratio	49.2
Smoking	35.7
Hypertension	17.9
Diabetes	9.9
Abdominal obesity	20.1
Psychosocial	32.5
Lack of daily fruit and vegetables	13.7
Lack of regular alcohol	6.7
Lack of regular physical activity	12.2

The inclusion of more variables would undoubtedly increase the accuracy of risk assessment, but also make it more complex. The presence of left ventricular hypertrophy in hypertensive individuals is a strong predictor of future risk but is rarely identified in primary care. Family history is a glaring omission but difficult to integrate. The Joint British Societies recommend multiplying the calculated 10-year cardiovascular risk by a factor of 1.5 where there is premature cardiovascular disease (<55 years in men and <65 years in women).

INTERHEART is a recent case-control study of 15 152 cases of myocardial infarction from 52 countries with 14 820 matched controls.[7] For each of nine major risk factors the study defined the increased risk of CHD expressed as the odds ratio (OR) and the population attributable risk (PAR). The PAR is a measure of the risk to a population of a risk factor based not only on the strength of the association of the risk factor but also its prevalence in that population. Individual PARs for the nine risk factors are shown in *Box 5.1* and together contributed 90.4% of the PAR for CHD, i.e. 90% of CHD in the world can be explained by nine conventional risk factors. The combined effect of the two most significant risk factors (the apo-B to apo-AI ratio and smoking) produces a PAR of 66.8%. Adding family history (OR 1.55) interestingly only shifts the PAR from 90.4 to 91.4%, suggesting that the risk of family history is largely mediated through the other risk factors.

There is much interest in the potential of emerging risk factors, particularly inflammatory markers such as CRP, and also new imaging techniques such as magnetic resonance, computed tomography and measurements of intimal thickness with carotid ultrasound. Computed tomography can detect and quantify coronary calcifications and define a calcium score which may be a useful marker of atherosclerosis in asymptomatic individuals. The results of prospective studies linking outcomes with coronary calcium scores are urgently needed to establish the role of this new technology.

5.6 At what threshold should treatment be initiated?

AFCAPS/TexCAPS (*see Q 8.4*) showed that using a statin in a primary prevention population whose 10-year risk of CHD was just 6% produced clinical benefit. The trial had to be terminated early when a relative risk reduction of 37% in CHD events was noted at the second interim analysis. The absolute reduction in events, however, was low and extrapolating the results into usual practice would mean a potentially untenable number of adults in most countries needing drug therapy, with limited gain.

An idea of the numbers identified by the latest threshold recommendations can be derived from a Scottish cohort of 3963 individuals aged 35–64 years.[8] Of this population, 8.5% were identified as needing

In primary prevention, the thresholds recommended by the major guidelines at which high risk is defined and lipid-lowering (and anti-hypertensive) therapy should be initiated are quite similar and are:

■ Joint British Societies: ≥20% 10-year cardiovascular event risk
■ European Society of Cardiology: ≥5% 10-year cardiovascular death risk
■ National Cholesterol Education Program (Adult Treatment Panel III): ≥20% 10-year CHD event risk.

It has already been noted that all three guidelines recommend automatic interventions in secondary prevention and diabetes.

Figure 5.1 shows the percentage risk thresholds recommended by the new Joint British Societies as a series of 'isobars'. The portion above the 20% 10-year cardiovascular event risk isobar is coloured red and represents high-risk individuals for whom interventions are recommended. Medium risk (10–20%) is coloured orange and low risk (<10%), green. Individuals at medium and low risk should follow good lifestyle habits but may choose to self-medicate, for example, with over-the-counter (OTC) statins if they fulfil the pharmacists' criteria (*see Q 9.18*).

secondary prevention interventions but, for primary prevention, a further 9.7% were identified at the 15% 10-year CHD risk level. A 15% 10-year CHD event risk is equivalent to a 10-year cardiovascular death risk of 5% (the European Society of Cardiology threshold) and this in turn is equivalent to a 20% 10-year cardiovascular event risk (the Joint British Societies' threshold). Given expanding age thresholds for primary prevention and the increasing absolute risk of cardiovascular disease with age, the numbers requiring treatment are set to expand enormously.

5.7 Can ethnicity be quantified?

The increased cardiovascular mortality seen in immigrant South Asian communities has been noted in several countries. The situation is complex, as cardiovascular risk varies among South Asian groups with significant differences in risk factors between Indians, Pakistanis and Bangladeshis. In the UK, CHD mortality is 40–50% higher than in age- and sex-matched Caucasians and the difference is increasing. This has led a number of commentators to advise multiplying the Framingham score by a factor of 1.4 to 1.5 to compensate for the increased risk. One community survey from south London confirmed that conventional Framingham-based assessment underestimated risk in South Asians and people of African origin in the management of hypertension. Instead of a 15% 10-year CHD risk threshold for intervention, the researchers suggested a 12% CHD 10-year threshold for South Asian people and 10% for those of African origin.[9]

PQ PATIENT QUESTIONS

5.8   How can I get my cardiovascular risk assessed?

It is important to remember that cardiovascular disease is multifactorial in origin. The most accurate risk assessments look at a range of cardiovascular risk factors, compare them mathematically to profiles of known risk and express the result as the percentage chance of a cardiovascular event over a period of time. Having a 20% 10-year cardiovascular event risk means 20 out of 100 people with the same risk will suffer a cardiovascular event, such as a heart attack or stroke, over the next 10 years. Halving the risk by treatment would result in 10 people being spared an event over 10 years.

Nowadays a range of health professionals are able to assess cardiovascular risk. Most commonly, this is done in primary care by GPs and nurses but there is overlap with hospital specialties. Some pharmacists have developed the same skills and 'over-the-counter' statins will only increase their number.

In the course of a cardiovascular risk assessment interview you can expect the following areas to be covered:

- Age
- Gender
- Ethnicity
- Personal medical history (especially high blood pressure or diabetes)
- Family history (especially events such as heart attacks, strokes or sudden death, and conditions such as angina, arterial disease, diabetes and high blood pressure or cholesterol)
- Smoking habit
- Alcohol intake
- Assessment of diet
- Assessment of physical activity.

You can expect measurements of height, weight and blood pressure (preferably a series of readings) and one or more blood tests to check levels of cholesterol, HDL-cholesterol and triglycerides. Triglycerides remain elevated for some hours after eating and you may be asked to fast (water and any regular medication only) for 12–14 hours if they are to be measured. Other blood tests, such as those assessing blood glucose, kidney, liver and thyroid function, may also be performed at the same time.

The results do not take long for the laboratory to perform and from them an estimate of the 10-year risk can be calculated and its significance interpreted by your healthcare adviser.

5.9   What is 'primary prevention'?

Primary prevention refers to the targeting of high-risk individuals with appropriate interventions before they develop a disease. In cardiovascular terms this chiefly means preventing the onset of heart attacks, angina and strokes. If you have no symptoms of these conditions you want to keep it that way.

5.10 What is 'secondary prevention'?

Secondary prevention refers to the prevention of further disease in an individual who already has the condition. In other words, if you have already been diagnosed with a cardiovascular disease you want to stop it getting worse.

5.11 What factors determine the level at which intervention is offered?

The guidelines which advise health professionals seek to strike a balance between the benefits and risks identified by the evidence base of clinical trials with what is achievable and what is affordable. At all levels of risk it is appropriate to follow a healthy lifestyle (*see Ch. 6*) and by developing thresholds for treatment the guidelines are really advising health professionals about the levels at which to start drug therapy.

The evidence of benefit for lipid-lowering drugs extends to very low levels of risk. However, implementing this evidence would mean drugs for the majority of adults and create a situation that no healthcare economy could sustain. Some individuals would be happy to take medication even if the absolute benefits were not very great, but many would not. In addition, the burdens of monitoring and fostering compliance would be too much for existing resources.

By choosing a threshold of, say, 20% 10-year cardiovascular event risk, the guidelines are identifying a cut-off point that may be deliverable within current structures of medical care (in terms of patient numbers and follow-up) as well as achieving a significant reduction in cardiovascular events within the population.

Treatment by diet and lifestyle

6.1	How do individuals change their habits?	79
6.2	How important is body shape?	80
6.3	What are the benefits of losing weight?	81
6.4	What is the effect of physical activity on lipids?	82
6.5	How does dietary fat affect lipids?	82
6.6	Does dietary cholesterol matter?	83
6.7	What is a cholesterol-lowering diet?	83
6.8	How effective is a cholesterol-lowering diet?	83
6.9	Does a cholesterol-lowering diet enhance the effect of medication?	84
6.10	What is a cardioprotective diet?	85
6.11	What are n-3 (omega-3) fatty acids?	86
6.12	What are the benefits of n-3 (omega-3) fatty acids?	87
6.13	What are plant stanols and sterols?	88
6.14	How do plant sterols work?	89
6.15	Are plant sterols safe?	89
6.16	Who should use plant sterols?	90
6.17	What is the role of soya?	90
6.18	What is the role of complex carbohydrates?	91
6.19	What is the 'portfolio' diet?	91
6.20	Is alcohol cardioprotective?	92
6.21	What are antioxidants?	93
6.22	Do antioxidants protect against heart disease?	93

PQ PATIENT QUESTIONS

6.23	How do I know if I am overweight?	94
6.24	How do I lose weight?	94
6.25	Is the 'Atkins' diet effective?	95
6.26	What are the most important dietary measures to prevent cardiovascular disease?	95
6.27	How do I stick to a cardioprotective diet?	96

6.28 What is the safe limit for alcohol and which type should I drink? 96

6.29 What other measures should I take to prevent cardiovascular disease? 97

6.1   How do individuals change their habits?

Traditional models of giving lifestyle advice are usually based on the explanation of risk and the giving of information, invariably delivered in a prescriptive and paternalistic manner. The recognition that patients only comply with about half of the advice they receive has led to a re-analysis of the processes of change involved in making lifestyle alterations. Prochaska and DiClemente's model[1] divides the process of change into five stages (*Box 6.1*).

The key for health professionals giving advice is to recognise the stage at which a patient presents and progress that individual through the cycle with appropriately timed motivation, information, goal setting and support. For example, intervening at the stage of preparation is much more likely to be successful than during the previous stages. The stages are cyclical and individuals may relapse several times before achieving success.

The value of changing lifestyle habits was demonstrated in the Lifestyle Heart Trial, first published in 1990.[2] In an era before the ubiquitous use of lipid-lowering drugs for the secondary prevention of coronary heart disease (CHD), Ornish et al showed that intensive lifestyle change (low fat vegetarian diet, moderate aerobic exercise, smoking cessation and psychological support) could reduce low density lipoprotein (LDL) cholesterol (by 37.2%) and angiographically reduce the progression of disease.[2]

Most recently, Neil and colleagues have described a reduction in non-cardiovascular deaths in treated patients with familial hypercholesterolaemia compared to the general population.[3] The risk of

---

BOX 6.1 Prochaska and DiClemente's stages of change

- *Precontemplation*: The individual is not interested in changing their 'risky' behaviour
- *Contemplation*: The individual is thinking about change but is ambivalent
- *Preparation*: There is an intention to take action and plans are made
- *Action*: Visible behaviour change begins
- *Maintenance*: Individuals work hard to prevent relapse

After DiClimente et al.[1]

cancer death was significantly reduced by 40%, largely due to a near-significant 50% reduction in gastrointestinal cancer and a highly significant 80% reduction in lung cancer. Lifestyle advice from healthcare professionals is likely to be responsible although individuals who see their family members affected by premature cardiovascular disease and death may improve their own health. Patients with familial hypercholesterolaemia (*see Qs 4.6–4.8*) are largely treated in lipid clinics where they will have received strong anti-smoking advice and also repeated dietary, weight control and exercise advice. Reduced fat intake, higher fibre intake and a better quality diet would be expected to influence their risk of gastrointestinal disease.

6.2 How important is body shape?

While individuals with high body mass index (BMI, *Fig. 6.1*) as a group have more CHD, the risk is heterogeneous and some individuals with raised BMI

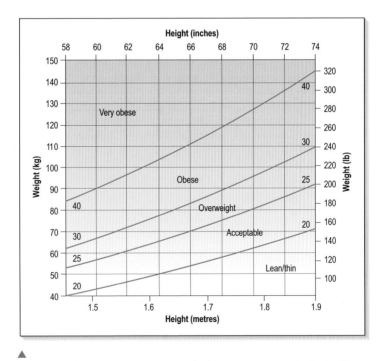

▲

Fig. 6.1 Obesity: relationship between height and weight. The numbers 20, 25, 30 and 40 represent the body mass index (BMI) at these curves. The BMI is weight (in kg) divided by height squared (in metres). (Adapted from Garrow,[4] with permission from Elsevier.)

have low cardiovascular risk. Raised BMI can result from a large muscle and bone mass and does not necessarily reflect adiposity. Interest has therefore focused on both the amount and distribution of adiposity as it has been known for more than 40 years that individuals with central obesity have higher risks of cardiovascular disease and diabetes than those in whom adiposity is more peripherally distributed.

Measurements of waist circumference have been shown by sophisticated scanning to correlate best with visceral adipose tissue and the risk of obesity-related complications (*Table 6.1*). Increased waist circumference is a feature of the metabolic syndrome (*see Q 4.3 and Box 1.1*) and Despres[5] has refined this further, describing the 'hypertriglyceridaemic waist phenotype' based on the observation that 80% of men with waist circumference >90 cm and hypertriglyceridaemia >2.0 mmol/L have metabolic disturbances which include hyperinsulinaemia, increased apolipoprotein B (apo-B), increased small dense LDL-cholesterol and their attendant cardiovascular risks.

6.3 What are the benefits of losing weight?

> The overconsumption of energy-dense diets, rich in fat and refined carbohydrate, coupled with reduced physical activity, are the reasons behind the growing trend towards obesity. Increasing BMI is associated with increasing blood pressure, total and LDL-cholesterol, apo-B, fasting triglycerides and fasting glucose and decreased high density lipoprotein (HDL) cholesterol and apolipoprotein AI.
>
> When overweight, reducing weight improves life expectancy, sleep apnoea, effort tolerance, musculoskeletal discomfort, physical appearance and self esteem. Blood pressure is reduced and there are favourable reverses in the lipid profile,[6] and in glucose in diabetes.

It has been calculated that a 10 kg weight loss in an individual with a baseline weight of 100 kg and co-morbidities would produce:

- ■ >20% fall in total mortality
- ■ >30% fall in diabetes-related death

TABLE 6.1 The risk of obesity-related complications by waist circumference

Risk of complications	Male waist circumference: cm (inches)	Female waist circumference: cm (inches)
Increased	>94 (37) (>90 Asian origin)	>80 (32)
Substantially increased	>102 (40)	>88 (35)

- >40% fall in obesity-related cancer death
- falls of 10 mmHg systolic and diastolic blood pressure
- 50% fall in fasting glucose if new diabetes
- 10% fall in total cholesterol
- 15% fall in LDL-cholesterol
- 30% fall in triglycerides
- 8% rise in HDL-cholesterol.

6.4 What is the effect of physical activity on lipids?

Numerous studies have shown that repeated, moderate amounts of aerobic activity result in reductions in total cholesterol, LDL-cholesterol and triglycerides and elevations in HDL-cholesterol. Plasma triglycerides show the greatest improvement and relate to increased activity of lipoprotein lipase in muscles and adipose tissue. The changes correlate with the degree of fitness achieved and the intensity of the activity such that very high levels of activity can reduce LDL-cholesterol by as much as 1 mmol/L and raise HDL-cholesterol significantly. For most sedentary individuals, current recommendations advising 30 minutes of moderate intensity physical activity on most days seems a sensible starting point but more exercise will confer greater benefit.

6.5 How does dietary fat affect lipids?

The bottom line is that high fat consumption increases cholesterol levels. High fat diets tend to be rich in saturated fats which increase total cholesterol, LDL-cholesterol and HDL-cholesterol as well as triglycerides. Furthermore, when in excess, the energy-dense nature of fat (9 kcal/g) contributes to calorie overconsumption and therefore the development of obesity and its compounding effects on the lipid profile.[7]

The total fat content of a diet, however, does not always correlate strongly with serum cholesterol as its different component fatty acids exert differing effects. For example, a diet rich in monounsaturated fatty acids (olive and rapeseed oil, most nuts, meat and avocados) reduces total and LDL-cholesterol and triglycerides while usually slightly raising HDL-cholesterol. Polyunsaturated fatty acids (sunflower, safflower and corn oils, most margarines, nuts and seeds) lower total cholesterol, LDL-cholesterol and triglycerides even more significantly but unfortunately reduce HDL-cholesterol.

Trans fatty acids (*see* Q 1.5 *and Fig. 1.1*) are the isomers of unsaturated fatty acids formed naturally in small amounts in ruminants and industrially in the hardening (by hydrogenation) of vegetable oils to produce margarine. Their straight chains make them behave like saturated fats. Responsible food manufacturers are now limiting their production.

Since the early 1970s a major reduction of total fat intake has seen reduced saturated and monounsaturated fatty acid consumption and increased use of polyunsaturates. Sadly, increased refined carbohydrate consumption coupled with reduced physical activity is driving the increasing prevalence of obesity.

6.6 Does dietary cholesterol matter?

Most individuals consume 300–500 mg cholesterol daily, chiefly from dairy products and meat. Some foods, especially eggs and shellfish, are particularly rich in cholesterol and many patients have been asked in the past to restrict their intake. It must be remembered that only 30–60% of dietary cholesterol is absorbed and as by far the most significant contribution to an individual's cholesterol level is from saturated fat, halving the intake of dietary cholesterol makes only a small impact on serum levels.

Epidemiological studies in healthy individuals have shown no correlation between egg consumption and cardiovascular disease. While rich in cholesterol (one large whole egg contains approximately 213 mg cholesterol), eggs contain only 5 g fat in total, two-thirds of which is unsaturated. The beneficial effects of the unsaturated components and additional antioxidants, folic acid and B vitamins probably offset any small adverse effect arising from the cholesterol content.

Food producers are often guilty of enhancing the credibility of their products by labelling them as 'low cholesterol'. This is misleading as what we eat to reduce cholesterol should be described as 'cholesterol lowering' not 'low cholesterol'.

6.7 What is a cholesterol-lowering diet?

The essence of the cholesterol-lowering diet is that total and saturated fat intakes are low, with part substitution by mono- and polyunsaturates and increased amounts of complex carbohydrate. There is broad agreement between consensus bodies and the results can be summarised as outlined in *Box 6.2*.

A major criticism of delivering dietary advice in this form is that for both health professionals and patients the recommendations are difficult to conceptualise and few possess the interpretative skills required to incorporate the recommendations into the practicalities of everyday eating.

6.8 How effective is a cholesterol-lowering diet?

In 1998, a meta-analysis of 19 randomised controlled trials showed only modest benefits for cholesterol-lowering diets.[8] With moderate intensity diets, a net reduction of only 3% in serum cholesterol is seen, rising to 6%

> **BOX 6.2 Example of a cholesterol-lowering diet**
> - Total fat: <30% of energy requirement
> - Saturated fat: <7–10%
> - Polyunsaturated fat: 7–10%
> - Monounsaturated fat: 10–15%
> - Cholesterol: <300 mg/day
> - Complex carbohydrates: 55% (especially vegetables, grains and legumes)
> - Protein: 15%
> - Total calories: reduce when weight loss is needed

with more rigorous regimes. Out of metabolic wards, where experimental diets achieve much more success, free-living individuals have less control over their diet and their compliance is tested by the amount and range of temptations on offer. In practice there is an enormous range in diet responsiveness and other studies show that changes in LDL-cholesterol vary from +5% to –40%.

The low fat, high complex carbohydrate diet described as the 'cholesterol-lowering diet' may not be suitable for everyone. The net effect is to reduce total and LDL-cholesterol but HDL-cholesterol is also reduced and triglycerides are elevated. In subjects with the metabolic syndrome (see Q 4.3) who already have low HDL-cholesterol and raised triglycerides this would not be ideal. A total low fat diet high in monounsaturates which reduce total and LDL-cholesterol, raise HDL-cholesterol and lower triglycerides would be more appropriate.

6.9 Does a cholesterol-lowering diet enhance the effect of medication?

The major improvements to lipid profiles often observed in the clinical trials of lipid-lowering medication tend to impress both health professionals and patients and lead to the false assumptions that a drug is all that is necessary and that the effect of diet is non-contributory. It should be remembered that the majority of drug trials establish an optimal dietary regime prior to introducing the study drug and that any benefits which accrue therefore are additional to the benefits of diet.

One study from America neatly showed the incremental benefit of an appropriate diet and simvastatin, demonstrating LDL-cholesterol reductions of 10.8% with a cholesterol-lowering diet, 29.7% with simvastatin and 40.5% when used together.[9]

6.10 What is a cardioprotective diet?

There has been much discussion concerning the optimal diet for the prevention of CHD. The Mediterranean diet (*Box 6.3*) is low in saturated fat and high in unsaturated fat, whereas Japanese diet is low in saturated fat but high in complex carbohydrates. Despite the differences, both diets are associated with the best life expectancies in the world.

The Mediterranean diet was tested in the CHD secondary prevention setting of the Lyon Diet Heart Study against 'a prudent western diet'.[10] After nearly 4 years, CHD deaths and non-fatal myocardial infarction were significantly reduced by 72% (albeit with wide confidence intervals). The benefits of the Mediterranean diet did not seem to be brought about by differences in traditional risk factors such as high blood pressure and cholesterol as comparison of the control and experimental groups at the end of the study showed few differences between them.

In recognition of the need for a more global approach to the dietary prevention of cardiovascular disease than the traditional cholesterol-lowering diet, the American Heart Association published revised dietary guidelines in 2000.[11] Key elements of the guidelines describing the cardioprotective diet are outlined in *Box 6.4*.

Labels such as 'low fat' and 'low salt' on processed foods can be misleading and those wishing to follow a cardioprotective diet should check food labels. A simple guide to food labelling is shown in *Table 6.2*.

BOX 6.3 Components of the Mediterranean diet

- Emphasis on fresh rather than processed foods
- High intake and variety of fruits, vegetables, legumes and grains – fresh fruit with meals as dessert
- High ratio of monounsaturated fatty acids to saturated fatty acids – olive oil as principal source of fat
- Moderate consumption of milk and dairy products – principally as cheese and yogurt
- Enhanced consumption of fish and poultry
- Low intake of red meat and meat products
- 0–4 egg yolks consumed weekly
- Alcohol consumption at moderate levels – typically wine with meal

BOX 6.4 American Heart Association dietary guidelines for the prevention of cardiovascular disease

■ Use foods and dietary patterns with broad health benefits:
  — fruit and vegetables five times a day
  — increased grain products (especially wholegrain cereals) six times a day
  — fat-free and low fat dairy products
  — fish twice a week
  — legumes, poultry and lean meat
■ Place greater emphasis on weight loss and obesity control:
  — match intake of energy to needs to prevent obesity and maintain a healthy body weight
  — limit intake of foods with high caloric value (especially sugars)
  — achieve a level of appropriate physical activity for weight maintenance or loss
■ Maintain a desirable blood cholesterol, lipoprotein profile and blood pressure:
  — limit intake of saturated fatty acids (<10%) and cholesterol (<300 mg/day)
  — minimise *trans* fats
  — substitute with grains, unsaturated fatty acids (especially from vegetables, fish, legumes and nuts)
  — limit salt to <6 g/day
  — limit alcohol to two drinks per day for men, one for women
  — maintain healthy body weight
  — emphasise fruit and vegetables and low fat products
■ Target special populations and higher risk subgroups with individual approaches:
  — older individuals, children, those with elevated LDL-cholesterol, pre-existing cardiovascular disease, diabetes mellitus, congestive heart failure or kidney disease.

After American Heart Association.[11]

6.11 What are n-3 (omega-3) fatty acids?

Fatty acids are formed from hydrocarbon chains with a terminal methyl group (*see Figs 1.1 and 1.2, and* Q 1.5). If a carbon/carbon double bond is present, the fatty acid is described as unsaturated. If more than one double bond is present, the fatty acid is polyunsaturated. The carbon of the terminal methyl group is called the omega carbon and the position of the first double bond is counted from this. Polyunsaturated fatty acids can be

TABLE 6.2 A simple guide to food labelling		
A lot		**A little**
20 g	Fat	3 g
5 g	Saturates	1 g
3 g	Fibre	0.5 g
10 g	Sugars	2 g
0.5 mg	Sodium	0.1 mg

divided into n-3 and n-6 fatty acids, meaning that the first unsaturated double bond is found at the third or the sixth carbon atom in the chain. The n-3 and n-6 polyunsaturated fatty acids have essential roles in the formation of prostaglandins and other prostanoid compounds.

Alpha linolenic acid is the principal n-3 polyunsaturated fatty acid occurring in the green tissue of plants and is converted in animals to small amounts of the longer chain n-3 fatty acids eicosapentaenoic acid (EPA) and docosahexaenoic acid (DHA). Alpha linolenic acid is found in greater concentration in soya bean, rapeseed and linseed oils and margarines and was a key component of the diet used in the Lyon Diet Heart Study.[10] Oily fish (e.g. sardines, pilchards, mackerel, herring, salmon, trout, halibut and tuna) concentrate EPA and DHA derived from alpha linolenic acid in phytoplankton and represent the best edible source of these n-3 polyunsaturates.

6.12 What are the benefits of n-3 (omega-3) fatty acids?

Attention was first drawn in 1927 to the low rates of CHD in fish-eating communities such as Greenland Inuits (Eskimos). Eventually, the differences were ascribed to the high levels of n-3 fatty acids derived from dietary fish, seal and whale meat. The Diet and Reinfarction Trial (DART) was a secondary prevention trial where the study group assigned to eating oily fish twice a week showed the surprising reduction in all-cause mortality of 29%.[12] The mechanisms for this benefit have been much debated and over 50 have been proposed.

Unlike n-6 polyunsaturates, which mainly reduce LDL-cholesterol and HDL-cholesterol, the most potent effect of n-3 polyunsaturates on the lipoprotein profile is to reduce triglyceride concentrations. LDL-cholesterol is usually little changed but HDL-cholesterol is raised. Changes in the lipid profile, however, would not account for the rapidity of benefit seen with n-3 fatty acids in secondary prevention and numerous studies support the hypothesis that they may have a membrane-stabilising effect, preventing malignant ventricular arrhythmias and, thereby, sudden death.[13] In addition, n-3 fatty acids have been shown to have beneficial effects on platelet aggregation, clotting factors, smooth muscle cells, inflammatory mediators, endothelial function, plasma viscosity and blood pressure.

The growing evidence for the cardioprotective benefit of n-3 fatty acids and the clear demonstration of their safety has led not only to their recommendation in modern dietary guidelines but also to the use of capsules of concentrated fish oil (*see Q 7.24*).

6.13 What are plant stanols and sterols?

Sterols (*Fig. 6.2*) are produced by both animals and plants and have analogous functions in maintaining cell membrane integrity. All sterols share the characteristic sterol ring but differences occur in the side chain at the C24 position and in the degree of saturation at the 5-alpha ring position. Confusingly, the term plant (or phyto-) sterol is used generically to describe both unsaturated sterols and saturated stanols together, as well as referring specifically to the unsaturated forms.

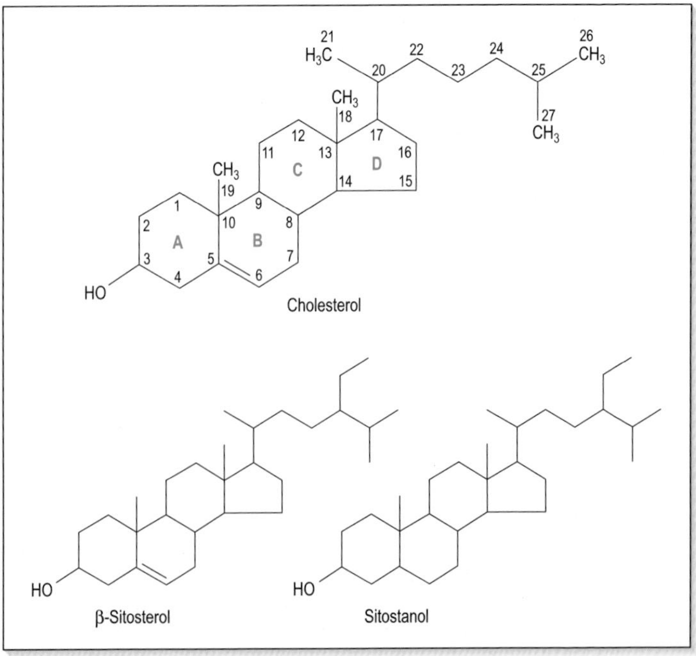

▲
Fig. 6.2 Sterol structures.

Whereas cholesterol is the sole sterol of mammalian cells, plants have evolved over 40 varieties, the commonest being β-sitosterol, campesterol and stigmasterol. Small amounts (150–400 mg/day) derive from vegetable oils, nuts, seeds, grains and legumes in the diet but over 50 years of research data show that larger quantities possess the capacity to significantly reduce serum cholesterol. The finding that, when esterified, plant sterols and stanols become soluble in other fats has led to the commercial development of a range of margarines, spreads and other vehicles now widely available to the general public. A meta-analysis of 41 trials of the efficacy of sterols and stanols suggests that a mean daily dose of 2 g of either will reduce LDL-cholesterol by 10.1% with no significant difference between the two.[14]

6.14   How do plant sterols work?

Foods enriched with plant sterols or stanols lower cholesterol by approximately halving the absorption of both dietary and biliary cholesterol. Hepatic cholesterol synthesis is increased but accelerated plasma clearance from the parallel upregulation of LDL-cholesterol receptors means the net effect is a reduction in both serum total and LDL-cholesterol. HDL-cholesterol and triglycerides are unaltered. Some formulations are less effective and only those with proven efficacy should be recommended.

Precisely how plant sterols and stanols achieve their reduction in intestinal cholesterol absorption is still not clear. Initially it was thought that competition with cholesterol within the mixed micelle was the explanation but the finding that plant stanols are just as effective when administered once a day, rather than with every meal when micelles are formed, has cast doubt on this explanation. Co-crystallisation with cholesterol to form insoluble compounds has been suggested, as has interference with gut lipase and esterase systems. Recently, the regulation of plant sterols has been found to involve members of the ABC transporter protein family (ATP binding cassette proteins). The intriguing finding that plant sterols increase the expression of ABC A-1, which has a regulatory role in the enterocyte promoting the efflux of absorbed cholesterol back into the gut lumen, may mean that specific effects on gut transporter proteins are the key.

6.15   Are plant sterols safe?

Despite the lack of long-term safety data, the regulatory authorities have approved the use of foods enriched with plant sterols and stanols for general consumption based on the likelihood that the balance between benefit and risk appears to be favourable.

Just like cholesterol, plant sterols are also potentially atherogenic and this is epitomised in the very rare disease familial phytosterolaemia, where premature atherosclerosis derives from heightened absorption of sitosterol.

Plant stanols do not pose this risk as they are virtually unabsorbed. About one in five million people is homozygous for this condition, now known to involve defects of the ABC G5 and G8 transporter systems and, for these individuals, plant sterol intake should be minimised. More importantly, about one in 1100 individuals is heterozygous for the condition and could theoretically be at risk from unsaturated plant sterol formulations. New research has shown, however, that this is not the case, with rapid hepatic clearance compensating for slightly increased absorption. In normal individuals unsaturated plant sterol preparations increase plasma sitosterol by 35% but as sitosterol is present in plasma at levels 100–1000 times lower than cholesterol, this is insignificant and more than offset by the reduction in LDL-cholesterol.

Plant sterols do not affect the levels of the fat-soluble vitamins A, D, E and K. They do not interfere with hormonal, biochemical or haematological processes and there are no drug interactions. Small reductions in alpha carotene and lycopene disappear when adjusted for LDL-cholesterol reduction (their carrier lipoprotein). Significant reductions of beta-carotene occur (8–19%) but these equate to seasonal variation, are offset by an extra portion of a carotenoid-containing fruit or vegetable and are of doubtful significance.

6.16 Who should use plant sterols?

Plant sterols demonstrate a consistent response irrespective of age, gender, background, diet or baseline cholesterol level and therefore have ubiquitous application in those who need cholesterol lowering. Similar LDL-cholesterol reduction has been shown in different patient subgroups such as those with CHD, diabetes or familial hypercholesterolaemia and in those already taking statins and fibrates. With statins, the adjuvant effect on LDL-cholesterol is greater than doubling the statin dose. More information is needed regarding combination use with bile acid sequestrants and ezetimibe (*see Ch. 7*).

A major outcome study is unlikely ever to happen given the difficulties involved in demonstrating an effect with an LDL-cholesterol reduction of 10%. Surrogate endpoint trials are awaited and animal models reassuringly confirm plaque reduction.

Due to expensive processing costs, plant sterol foods are expensive and the cost is borne by the patient. There is a tendency to minimise the amount of plant sterol used and this represents a challenge for the supportive health professional. Manufactures publish clear instructions on product labels to optimise daily intake.

6.17 What is the role of soya?

Soy protein intakes of up to 55 g/day have been one of the explanations put forward for the low rates of CHD in Japan. Soy protein comes from the soya bean and can be used to replace other sources of animal or plant protein in the diet. Soy protein may be consumed as whole beans, soy nuts, soy milk, yoghurt and cheese, in traditional foods such as tofu, miso and tempeh or, after processing, as an enormous variety of meat and poultry analogues.

> In those with higher baseline cholesterol, 25 g of soy protein per day, as part of a diet low in saturated fat and cholesterol, reduces LDL-cholesterol by about 6%.[15] Larger reductions are obtained when soy protein is substituted completely for animal protein due to the additional reduction in saturated fat. There seems to be no effect in individuals with low cholesterol.

The cholesterol-lowering properties of the soya bean seem to depend both on soy protein (which has been shown to upregulate LDL-cholesterol receptors) and the additional effect of soy isoflavones. Soy isoflavones are also essential constituents of the soya bean and are weakly oestrogenic, reducing LDL-cholesterol and raising HDL-cholesterol.

In 1999 the US Food and Drug Administration (FDA) approved the claim of incorporating 25 g/day of soy protein into the diet to reduce CHD.

6.18 What is the role of complex carbohydrates?

Dietary patterns rich in complex carbohydrates are associated with a decreased risk of cardiovascular disease. Part of the effect results from the actions of insoluble fibre which promotes satiety by slowing gastric emptying and helps to control calorie intake and therefore weight. In addition, certain soluble fibres (e.g. oat bran, psyllium, pectin and guar gum) in feasible amounts have a small LDL-cholesterol lowering quality of about 2–3%, which is about the same as substituting unsaturated fats for saturated fats.[16]

Whether they work by promoting satiety or by more specific actions, complex carbohydrates are an integral part of the balanced diet. Modern guidelines emphasise the role of wholegrains such as wheat, corn, oats, barley, rye and rice as they contain ideal mixtures of complex carbohydrates, vitamins, trace minerals and fibre.

6.19 What is the 'portfolio' diet?

In 2002, Jenkins et al published a small study examining the potential effect of combining plant sterols, soy protein and soluble fibre on blood lipids in 13 hypercholesterolaemic patients already consuming a low fat diet.[17] The rationale was that, by using a portfolio approach with a range of

TABLE 6.3 One-day menu plan (200 kcal) 'portfolio' diet

Breakfast	Lunch	Dinner	Snacks
Oat bran, orange, psyllium, oat bran bread, plant sterol margarine, double fruit jam, soy milk	Vegetarian chilli, oat bran bread, plant sterol margarine, soy slices, tomato, orange	Vegetable curry, soy burger, beans, barley, okra, aubergine, cauliflower, onions, red pepper	Almonds, psyllium, soy milk, soy yoghurt, double fruit jam

cholesterol-lowering components, each with differing modes of action, this would produce greater cholesterol reduction than traditional approaches. The foods were all available in supermarkets and health food stores, and a typical one-day menu plan is shown in *Table 6.3*.

Remarkably, after just 4 weeks, LDL-cholesterol was reduced by 29% (± 2.7%). A second study, with 46 subjects consuming a similar vegan diet, not only replicated the findings but also showed equivalent LDL-cholesterol reduction to the use of a statin and beneficial changes in the inflammatory marker C-reactive protein (CRP).[18]

6.20 Is alcohol cardioprotective?

The U-shaped relationship between alcohol consumption and overall mortality was first recognised in the 1920s. More than 60 studies have shown that people who drink small amounts of alcohol regularly have less CHD than non-drinkers and those who drink more heavily. Large cohort studies have consistently shown that moderate alcohol consumption of one to two drinks a day is associated with a relative risk reduction of CHD death of approximately one-third.

About half of the benefit of moderate alcohol consumption is mediated through a rise in HDL-cholesterol. One or two drinks a day raise HDL-cholesterol by 12% but with increasing consumption, hepatic cell death may cause HDL-cholesterol to fall. Like any source of carbohydrates, alcohol produces a concomitant rise in triglyceride production and very low density lipoprotein (VLDL) secretion and this offsets the effect of a rise in HDL-cholesterol. A fatty liver can ensue and in some individuals with impaired triglyceride catabolism, very high levels of triglycerides are seen with potentially life-threatening pancreatitis. Raised triglyceride levels are a common marker of excess alcohol consumption, particularly in men.

The remainder of alcohol's beneficial action derives largely from its antithrombotic effects. Fibrinogen and tissue factor are reduced and there are favourable actions on plasminogen activation and platelet aggregation.

6.21 What are antioxidants?

Oxidation and reduction reactions are key features of normal cellular processes but result in the generation of reactive oxygen species (ROS) such as the free radical, superoxide (O_2^-). Exogenous sources of ROS include ionising radiation, cigarette smoke, pollutants, various toxins and poisons. ROS molecules are powerful oxidants and in seeking an electron to stabilise their outer ring are responsible for harmful effects on the body, such as the oxidisation of LDL-cholesterol, injury to cell membranes and damage to proteins and DNA. Reactive oxygen species are therefore implicated in the processes of cardiovascular disease, cancer and ageing.

A complex system of antioxidants exists to counteract the excessive effects of ROS and work by enzyme systems, redox pathways or structural conformations capable of neutralising the ROS charge. Many of the enzyme systems are reliant on trace elements such as selenium, manganese, copper and zinc. Antioxidants that diffuse ROS charge include tocopherols, ubiquinol, carotenoids, flavonoids, ascorbate, urate and thiols.

Much interest has focused on the possibility that high intake of antioxidant vitamins (particularly vitamins E, C and beta-carotene) might offset ageing and disease and in affluent populations, vitamin supplementation is common. Herbert has said that 'Americans excrete the richest urine in the world'.

6.22 Do antioxidants protect against heart disease?

Epidemiological studies suggest that differences in antioxidant status are related to the risk of cancer and cardiovascular disease. Populations with low intakes of fruit and vegetables (which are good sources of antioxidant vitamins and trace minerals) have consistently shown increased risks of developing heart disease and cancer. The problem with these studies is that it is difficult to separate the benefits of antioxidants from the effects of other parallel behaviour patterns and influences that could be confounding.

Controlled clinical trials of antioxidant supplementation are one answer but in the main have been inconsistent and mostly negative. The Heart Protection Study showed no benefit in using an antioxidant 'cocktail' of three supplements (vitamin E 600 mg, vitamin C 250 mg and beta-carotene 20 mg) compared to placebo, each taken by over 10 000 patients for over 5 years. Critics have pointed out that the choice of supplements and their doses may not have been ideal and that the trial may have been too short but the study has dealt a body blow to the idea that vitamin supplements can prevent heart disease.

The balanced view is that we should maintain a high intake of fruit and vegetables without supplementation by pills. The antioxidant system may depend on complex synergistic mechanisms to be effective. Without doubt, more will be heard of the antioxidant story and new research has already shown potential benefits in slowing the progression of macular degeneration and reducing cognitive decline.

PQ PATIENT QUESTIONS

6.23 How do I know if I am overweight?

Exactly where healthy weight ends and unhealthy weight begins has been a matter of much debate. The body mass index (BMI) is the measurement most often used to relate an individual's weight to their height and can be identified using simple charts (*see Fig. 6.1*) or the equation:

$$\text{BMI (kg/m}^2) = \text{weight (kg)} \div \text{height (m}^2)$$

The World Health Organization defines normal weight as a BMI of 18.5–24.9 kg/m², overweight as >25 kg/m² and obesity as >30 kg/m². While it is recognised that individuals with high BMI as a group have an increased risk of complications, not all individuals with the same BMI will suffer the same fate. Raised BMI can result from a large mass of muscle or bone and does not automatically reflect a high body fat content. More and more, health professionals are targeting individuals with increased abdominal girth, recognising that this is a much better correlate of body fat than BMI. Simple measurements of the ratio of waist to hip size or (even better) just waist circumference are increasingly relevant (*see Q 6.2*).

6.24 How do I lose weight?

There is no overweight individual with hyperlipidaemia whose lipid levels would not be improved by losing weight. The most common strategy remains the calorie-controlled diet and this is based on the premise that losing 1 kg of excess weight demands an energy deficit of 7000 kcal. If the weight loss is required over 1 week, then this means a deficit of 1000 kcal per day. As the average man requires 2500 kcal/day and the average woman 2100 kcal/day all individuals should lose weight on a diet of 1000 kcal/day and this is confirmed in controlled studies. Sadly, calorie counting is often ineffective as it is complex, demands meticulous measurement and recording, is often poorly tailored to the individual and the facility to deceive is high.

Behaviour modification techniques which recognise the preparedness of an individual to change (*see Q 6.1*) are more successful and are often used by dieting groups and health professionals to improve compliance. Improving self-esteem, controlling eating cues and body image dissatisfaction, providing contingency plans and social and psychological support or simply eating more slowly all work. The individual should:

- understand the benefits of weight loss (*see* Q 6.3)
- critically analyse their diet (food diaries are helpful here)
- construct a coherent plan (above all, *eat smaller portions*)
- increase physical activity (activity loses fat more than muscle)
- set targets that are realistic and attainable
- enlist support (surveys show that for both men and women, support and follow-up are critical in maintaining long-term weight loss).

6.25 Is the 'Atkins' diet effective?

Since 1973, when Dr Robert Atkins first published his theories, more than 10 million copies of his books have been sold. The high protein/low carbohydrate approach flies in the face of conventional guidance and has gained much popular appeal but evidence of benefit is more anecdotal than scientific. One recent small study showed superior initial weight loss on the Atkins diet but no difference after 1 year when compared to a traditional low fat, calorie-controlled approach.[19] The initial success is likely to be due to the breakdown of the body's carbohydrate stores and loss of fluid but there may also be a novelty effect in trying a new diet. At 1 year, the drops in total and LDL-cholesterol usually seen with weight loss were negated by the high fat intake but a rise in HDL-cholesterol and a drop in triglycerides were significant.

Adherence to a diet is a critical issue in long-term weight loss and maintenance. In this trial, adherence to the Atkins diet was poor and over a third of patients dropped out. A low carbohydrate diet requires the breakdown of fats in the body for energy and this releases chemicals known as ketones which make your breath smell and induce weakness, nausea and dehydration.

In the long term, there are theoretical concerns about the safety of the Atkins diet. Heart disease, stroke and cancer may all be promoted by the high fat, low fibre, low fruit and vegetable, low vitamin regime. Chronic high protein consumption could aggravate kidney disease and low calcium levels might impair bone health.

On the basis of current evidence, as the safety of the Atkins diet has not been established and aspects directly contradict well-founded dietary advice, it cannot be recommended.

6.26 What are the most important dietary measures to prevent cardiovascular disease?

Many health professionals are poorly equipped to interpret dietary recommendations with the consequence that important messages are often badly delivered and for many patients the complexity and negativity of the advice can be off-putting.

Current guidance can be distilled into ten hot tips!

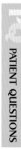

1. Enjoy a wide variety of fresh, not processed foods.
2. Be a healthy weight for your height.
3. Eat plenty of fruit, vegetables and salad.
4. Eat fish twice a week.
5. Base meals and snacks around starchy carbohydrates like potatoes, bread, cereals, rice and pasta.
6. Eat a diet low in fat, especially in saturated and *trans* fats.
7. Substitute saturated and *trans* fats with monounsaturated and polyunsaturated fats.
8. Choose lean meat, poultry, legumes, nuts, soya and low fat dairy foods.
9. Eat less salt.
10. Maintain sensible alcohol limits.

6.27 How do I stick to a cardioprotective diet?

No diet that is dull, uninteresting or unpalatable will secure compliance and heart-healthy diets have this unfounded reputation. Sticking to the right diet entails:

- making sure you enjoy your food
- understanding the components of the balanced, cardioprotective diet
- making sure you eat a wide variety of foods with different flavours, textures and colours; traditional recipes can be adapted to healthier versions
- developing a 'cardioprotective kitchen', stocked with largely fresh, heart-healthy ingredients and equipped to cook with healthier techniques
- involving the whole family; the cardioprotective diet is appropriate for life and is a powerful model for children
- checking food labels (a simple guide is shown in *Table 6.2*)
- maintaining the principles of the cardioprotective diet when eating away from the home.

6.28 What is the safe limit for alcohol and which type should I drink?

Studies have shown that drinking a moderate amount of alcohol on a daily basis is good for heart health (*see* Q 6.20). There seems to be little benefit beyond one to two drinks a day as, with increasing consumption, the risk of liver disease, high blood pressure, heart and stroke disease, various cancers, accidents and violent death all increase. The current consensus weekly limits of 21 units for men and 14 units for women seem eminently sensible.

You can work out the exact number of units in a drink by multiplying the volume (in mL) by the percentage 'abv' (alcohol by volume – found on the label) and dividing it by 1000. For example, the number of units in a 330 mL bottle of lager with a 5% abv is:

$$330 \times 5 = 1650 \div 1000 = 1.7 \text{ units.}$$

Similarly, the number of units:

- in a 440 mL can of extra strong lager (9% abv) is 4
- in a 250 mL (large) glass of wine (12% abv) is 3 (a full bottle has 9 units!).
- in a 25 mL (pub measure) of spirits (37.5% abv) is 1.

Diluting drinks by adding water or mixers, of course, makes no difference to their alcohol content.

The amount of column inches devoted to identifying the optimum amount of alcohol is vast yet comfortably exceeded by the coverage accorded to discussing which type of alcohol is the most protective. The benefits of red wine, in particular, are commonly extolled by many health professionals and plausible explanations involving other bioactive constituents abound. The bottom line is that, across the totality of the studies, there is no evidence that any particular alcoholic drink has any greater effect than any other with the same amount of ethanol. In short, it is the alcohol that counts.

6.29 What other measures should I take to prevent cardiovascular disease?

About a fifth of heart disease deaths and about a quarter of all deaths are directly attributable to smoking. The World Health Report of 2002 notes that 3% of the disease burden in developed countries and up to a quarter of heart disease deaths are associated with physical inactivity. Therefore:

- *Smokers should stop smoking*: Surveys show that two-thirds of smokers would like to give up their habit and modern counselling techniques allied to nicotine replacement therapy with or without bupropion can achieve 12-month quit rates of up to 22.5%.
- *Increase physical activity*: Current advice is to be 'moderately active' for 30 minutes, preferably every day. Brisk walking epitomises moderate activity, being exertion sufficient to induce mild sweating and breathlessness.

For many individuals at high risk, drug therapy is indicated and this is covered in *Chapter 7*. The informed patient should be aware of available therapies, their potential benefits and hazards and the target levels to which risk factors should be modified. Developing a therapeutic alliance with health professionals will ensure an individual adds the benefits of modern preventative interventions to a healthy lifestyle.

Drug treatments for dyslipidaemia

7

STATINS

7.1 How do statins work?   101

7.2 Who should receive a statin?   102

7.3 Who else may gain from statin therapy?   103

7.4 Should cholesterol be measured before statin initiation?   104

7.5 Who should not receive a statin?   105

7.6 What are the side effects of statins?   106

7.7 Why does myopathy occur?   107

7.8 What safety monitoring should be undertaken?   108

7.9 How should myalgia be managed?   108

7.10 What action should be taken for raised transaminases?   109

7.11 What drug interactions are seen with statins?   109

7.12 Are all statins the same?   110

7.13 Do all statins have the same risk of side effects?   111

7.14 If adverse effects occur with one statin, is it worth switching to another?   113

7.15 Is it best to treat to target or use the doses used in clinical trials?   114

7.16 What are the implications of a poor response to treatment?   115

FIBRATES

7.17 How do fibrates work?   115

7.18 What are the indications for a fibrate?   115

7.19 What are the side effects of fibrates?   116

7.20 Are all fibrates the same?   116

OTHER PHARMACOLOGICAL TREATMENTS

7.21 How does ezetimibe work?   117

7.22 What is the role of ezetimibe?   118

7.23 What are the side effects of ezetimibe?   118

7.24 What is the role of omega-3 fish oil capsules?   119

7.25 What is the role of nicotinic acid?   119

7.26 Why is nicotinic acid not used more widely?   119

7.27 What is the role of bile acid sequestrants? 120

7.28 Why are resins used so much less now? 120

7.29 What are the roles of metformin and the thiazolidinediones? 121

7.30 When is combination therapy required? 121

7.31 Which drug combinations are preferred? 122

ALTERNATIVE TREATMENTS

7.32 What radical therapy is available? 123

PATIENT QUESTIONS

7.33 What alternative therapies are available for raised cholesterol and blood fats? 124

7.34 Do drugs cure the problem? 124

7.35 At what time of day should lipid-lowering medication be taken? 125

7.36 Do lipid-lowering drugs cause impotence? 125

7.37 How do I know if lipid-lowering drugs are being effective? 126

7.38 What other drugs are advised in patients at high cardiovascular risk? 126

STATINS

7.1 How do statins work?

Statins are a group of drugs that reduce the synthesis of cholesterol by competitively inhibiting the enzyme 3-hydroxy-3-methyl-glutaryl coenzyme-A (HMG-CoA) reductase, thus blocking a key step in the synthesis of cholesterol from HMG-CoA to mevalonate (*see Fig. 1.5*). Around 90% of the flux through this pathway is to cholesterol, but 10% of the products are diverted to side routes. The geranyl, farnesyl and geranylgeranyl pyrophosphate compounds have 10, 15 and 20 carbons respectively. The latter two compounds are attached to a number of other compounds and proteins, and these farnesylated and geranylgeranylated compounds have a number of modulatory roles. For instance, they may help modify the pathways that lead to expression of inflammatory mediators and cytokines, so that potential arterial wall inflammation would be limited. This would be a possible 'pleiotropic' effect of a statin, i.e. an effect that was not directly due to LDL-cholesterol lowering. The effect might require substantial statin dose, above that for LDL lowering, and outcome evidence on cardiovascular disease (CVD) events has not been demonstrated in clinical trials.

While statins can reduce cholesterol synthesis in many tissues, their prime site of action is in the liver (*Fig. 7.1*). Cholesterol synthesis in the liver leads to the secretion of very low density lipoproteins (VLDLs) and low density lipoproteins (LDLs), and is also needed for bile acid production. If liver synthesis is partly inhibited then there is upregulation of the number of receptors on liver cells for LDLs, an increased uptake of plasma LDLs to maintain cholesterol availability within liver cells, and thus a fall in blood cholesterol values.

Statins do not sufficiently block cholesterol synthesis to cause too low a cholesterol level, nor to block other products that come from the same synthetic pathway. Adrenal and gonadal steroids are synthesised from cholesterol, but neither synthesis of cholesterol in these glands nor levels of blood cholesterol to be taken up by the glands are reduced enough to influence the synthesis of these steroid hormones. Indeed it is possible that modest changes in some of the side products from the cholesterol synthetic pathway may reduce the inflammatory processes that partly characterise arterial atherogenesis.

The effects of statins can be augmented by steps to reduce cholesterol absorption from the gut, for if there is less cholesterol reaching the liver then there is a further increase in hepatic cell LDL receptor expression and LDL uptake. Reducing dietary cholesterol is

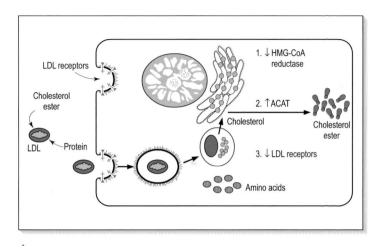

▲

Fig. 7.1 Cholesterol metabolism within cells. Low density lipoproteins (LDLs) carry cholesterol in the blood to tissues which are able to take up the LDLs if needed. Cells synthesise LDL receptors and place these in the cell membrane when cholesterol is needed. The LDL particle binds to the receptor, the complex is internalised and free cholesterol is liberated in the cell. As the cell becomes replete with cholesterol in this way the cell: (1) esterifies and stores any excess cholesterol not used, (2) switches off the cell's own cholesterol production and (3) reduces the recycling of LDL receptors into the cell membrane to limit further cholesterol absorption. ACAT, acyl coenzyme A cholesterol acyltransferase; HMG-CoA, 3-hydroxy-3-methyl-glutaryl coenzyme-A.

therefore beneficial, and there are two groups of drugs that can further help. These are the bile acid sequestrants (*see Q 7.27*) which cause the liver to redirect cholesterol to bile salt synthesis, and the cholesterol absorption inhibitor, ezetimibe (*see Q 7.21*).

7.2 Who should receive a statin?

Statins are indicated for the treatment of hypercholesterolaemia or mixed hyperlipidaemia where the predominant rise is in cholesterol rather than triglycerides. Statins should be accompanied by full dietary and lifestyle advice, and secondary causes of hyperlipidaemia should have been excluded or treated.

Statins should be prescribed to those whose coronary heart disease (CHD) risk is sufficient to warrant treatment and where hypercholesterolaemia is a component of that risk.

The benefits of statin therapy are substantial, the side effects low, the serious adverse events rare, and evidence for benefit extends to low levels of cholesterol and LDL-cholesterol. Cholesterol levels fall fully well within 1 month and outcome benefits begin to be apparent within 3–12 months, but treatments should be considered lifelong or long term. Use is determined not by chronological age but by biological age, and individuals at sufficiently high risk should be treated if they have a reasonable likelihood of life expectancy of 3 years or more.

All patients with existing macrovascular disease – cardiac, cerebral and peripheral – should be treated. Familial hypercholesterolaemia (FH) has such a high cardiovascular risk that all patients require treatment. It is also now considered that diabetes has sufficiently high risk to be considered a CHD risk equivalent, and should be managed as secondary prevention. Those without disease should be treated if their cardiovascular (cardiac plus cerebral) risk exceeds 20% over the following 10 years (equivalent to a CHD risk exceeding 15%/10 years). These risks have been calculated from the Joint British Societies' guidelines for the (primary) prevention of CHD,[1] either using a computer program or using the charts (see back pages of the *British National Formulary*). The updated, revised charts from the new Joint British Societies' guidelines are shown in *Figure 5.1*. These demonstrate treatment need for primary prevention when a person is above a 20% risk of a cardiovascular event over the next 10 years (equivalent to a 15% CHD risk over 10 years). This risk is calculated from the gender and age of the patient together with smoking, blood pressure and cholesterol/HDL-cholesterol ratio. The charts are not for use in those who already have vascular disease, diabetes or an inherited lipid disorder, in all of whom treatment will normally be required (*see Q 10.8*). The new charts are also available from the BMJ web pages (http://bmj.bmjjournals.com/cgi/content/full/320/7236/705).

The recommendations in the Joint British Guidelines[1] were endorsed by the Department of Health in both the National Service Framework (NSF) for coronary heart disease and the NSF for diabetes. They have also been included in the new primary care contract for general practitioners – the GMS contract. The GMS contract is still using the 1998 guidelines, which are now quite conservative, and has set a low standard of 60% for the percentage of secondary prevention patients who should meet a target of cholesterol <5 mmol/L. The criteria and standards in the GMS contract are likely to be reviewed in 2006.

7.3 Who else may gain from statin therapy?

In 2004, the first statin became available directly from the pharmacist for suitable patients as the first drug to be available for chronic use (*see also Q 9.16*). Unlike current pharmacy medicines available to the public, statins do require the pharmacist to ensure that patients at high risk, with other conditions or on other medications, will be referred back to their doctors. The pharmacist will also ensure that an 'over-the-counter' (OTC) statin supply is given only to those at appropriate moderate cardiovascular risk. The target groups are those individuals likely to have a cardiovascular risk of 10–20% over 10 years without contraindications to statin treatment. They are males aged 45–55 years and females of 55 years and above who have one other risk factor (obesity, tobacco use, poor family history, Asian/ethnic risk). Males of 55 years and above are eligible without any additional risk factor. The first agent, simvastatin (which is now off-patent), is available at the low, starting dose of 10 mg daily.

Cholesterol measurement prior to, and on treatment is encouraged, and, if cholesterol remains significantly raised, such individuals should be encouraged to visit their primary care team. Indeed, it is likely that individuals willing to purchase their long-term treatment will wish to observe their pre-treatment and on-treatment cholesterol values to ensure there is a sufficiency of response and that inadequately managed individuals are recognised. This would be the authors' strong views. At these levels of risk there are significant benefit-to-risk gains as statin risks are very low, but individuals who choose to purchase their own statin over the pharmacy counter need to recognise that rather larger numbers of individuals will need to be treated to prevent an event than would usually be considered within the National Health Service. However, and depending on the price of the statin, this may still approach the levels at which standard cost-effectiveness levels for intervention are reached.

Other individuals will not wish to take this route – they may feel that the taking of their first medicine will be 'converting them from a person into a patient'. For some there are clearly psychological and other factors where they would feel better without treatment. At these lower risk levels such decisions are entirely appropriate.

In the new JBS guideline charts (*see Fig. 5.1*) there is an amber-coloured area where cardiovascular risk is between 10 and 20% over 10 years, where treatment benefits are clearly present, and outweigh the small side effect risk. These levels are those where pharmacist-controlled availability would be appropriate.

7.4 Should cholesterol be measured before statin initiation?

In primary CVD prevention, for the most effective management and to assess responses, it would be appropriate to measure not only cholesterol but also a fasting lipid profile. Furthermore, secondary causes of hyperlipidaemia of renal, hepatic and thyroid disease should be excluded, and a fasting glucose would be appropriate. Patients with significant hypertriglyceridaemia may need different or additional management.

In secondary prevention it is now usual practice to commence a statin when an individual has a random cholesterol elevated on admission to the coronary care unit. The cholesterol level tends to fall (and at times significantly) 24 hours after an acute event, and therefore may not be a fully reliable measurement, whereas triglycerides tend to rise.

> The important issue is to ensure that a further set of measurements, ideally a fasting lipid profile, is taken after treatment has been initiated to ensure targets are being reached. Statins have full effect by 1–3 weeks, while after an acute illness a delay of to 2–3 months is appropriate to allow lipid levels to stabilise fully.

7.5   Who should not receive a statin?

> ■ Statins should not be given routinely to individuals who do not have some significant cardiovascular risk.
> ■ Statins should not be given to children, except in rare circumstances of familial hypercholesterolaemia with poor family risk, and then only under the advice of a specialist in lipid disorders.
> ■ Statins should not be given in pregnancy, and women are advised to discontinue their statin from conception planning until the end of breast feeding. Pregnancies on statins have been recorded without evidence of teratogenicity, but other studies have suggested an increased risk (*see also Q 10.5*).
> ■ Statins should not be given to the rare individuals with a prior major adverse event to a statin without careful consideration and usually with specialist advice. The major but very rare concern is of acute myositis and rhabdomyolysis, thought to occur about once per 50 000 patient-years of treatment. Consideration needs to be given to concomitant renal or hepatic disease, exclusion of untreated hypothyroidism, and other pharmacotherapy.

At the present time benefit is demonstrated in randomised clinical trials down to a cardiovascular risk of below 10%/10 years, although statin acquisition costs may limit National Health Service provision to patients at 20%/10 year CVD risk and above. With generic statins the cost–benefit will fall and many individuals in the 10–20%/10 year risk (and even below) may become eligible. In the short term such moderate risk individuals may contemplate purchasing their own OTC low-dose (simva)statin.

Statins are variously and to variable extent metabolised through the cytochrome P450 system in the liver, the major route for drug detoxification and removal (*see Table 7.1*). Statins metabolised via the P450

3A4 pathway (atorvastatin, simvastatin, lovastatin and previously cerivastatin) are potentially more likely to have drug interactions as other drugs are also metabolised through this route, while others through P450 2C9 and 2C19 (fluvastatin, rosuvastatin) or not through P450 (pravastatin) may have less interaction risk. Risks rise with higher statin doses, and in the 3A4 system the conazoles, ciclosporin, erythromycin and protease inhibitors are examples of drugs with potential interaction.[2]

 There were very particular issues with the fibrate gemfibrozil, leading to the withdrawal of cerivastatin in August 2001 (*www.fda.gov*), but other fibrates such as fenofibrate seem not to have such a predilection. The cerivastatin–gemfibrozil interaction seems not to be fully accounted for by their interactions through the 3A4 pathway alone, and other drug clearance mechanisms may play a role. That there are also pathways other than 3A4 is indicated by myositis risk with some statins that are not 3A4 metabolised. Risks are higher in the older female with a small body mass.

7.6   What are the side effects of statins?

 In the many double-blind, randomised, placebo-controlled trials of statins the side effect rates have been very low, without significant differences from adverse-event withdrawal between verum and placebo groups.

The main side effect of statins is myopathy, which is uncommon. This is associated with a rise in the muscle enzyme, creatinine (phospho)kinase (CPK, CK). Acute myositis is associated with a rise in CK to >10 times the upper limit of normal. If this progresses without drug withdrawal it can lead to severe muscle damage (rhabdomyolysis) and muscle breakdown leading to renal failure and rarely death. The CK value can be very variable even in normal individuals not on any treatments, and can rise markedly with energetic exercise, especially if this is unaccustomed. Random CK measurements in asymptomatic individuals are therefore rarely helpful and should be avoided in routine patient treatment. In asymptomatic individuals an isolated rise in CK up to five times, or even 10 times, the upper limit of normal can be acceptable.

There are individuals taking a statin who experience muscle discomfort without CK change. Other statins, and at low dose, can be tried. The risk–benefit in a patient at high CVD risk, and the severity of the symptoms can be discussed with the patient, but some will need treatments other than a statin. The symptoms are of a generalised muscle discomfort, pain, weakness or tenderness, rather akin to the symptoms on the first days of 'acute influenza'. Localised muscle group symptoms, cramps in the calves and joint-related symptoms are not indicative of a statin relationship.

Liver enzymes can also rise occasionally with statin therapy although this is very rarely of significance if there is not severe underlying liver disease. It is recommended therefore that liver transaminases are checked prior to statin initiation. In asymptomatic individuals an isolated rise in alanine aminotransferase (ALT) up to three times the upper limit of normal can be acceptable. Where liver enzymes are abnormal prior to statin initiation the cause of the liver disorder should be identified. Levels of ALT should then be monitored to ensure major deteriorations do not occur. One of the relatively common difficulties is in higher risk patients with accompanying hypertriglyceridaemia, obesity, glucose intolerance or diabetes in whom fatty infiltration of the liver is often associated with mild liver enzyme disturbance, known as non-alcoholic fatty liver diseases (NAFLD). Care should be exercised in patients indulging in major alcohol excess.

While some patients may note non-specific symptoms (e.g. gastrointestinal), which may or may not be treatment related, it is then appropriate to try an alternative statin.

Recently moderate tubular (not glomerular) proteinuria has been found with most statins (and also small amounts of microscopic haematuria), predominantly with high-dose rosuvastatin. At present this seems to be due to HMG-CoA reductase inhibition in the renal tubule, related to the high affinity binding of rosuvastatin to the enzyme. This seems to limit tubular reabsorption of proteins. Currently it does not seem to influence long-term renal function. This area is being closely observed.

Other concerns surrounding OTC statins are outlined in *Box 9.3*.

7.7　Why does myopathy occur?

 Exact reasons for myopathy are not fully understood. It is clear that it is statin-dose related, being rarer at low doses, and increasing somewhat at higher doses. It is also clear that a patient who has been symptomatic with one statin will often, but not always, have symptoms with others. It is more common in those with other significant medical illnesses, in women, in those with a small body mass and those more elderly.

Often there may be contributory factors, of which other drug therapy is common. Where drugs are metabolised in the liver through the same pathway as the statin being used, there is considerably higher risk of drug interaction, leading in some cases to major elevations in the circulating statin drug level. High plasma levels of statin are myotoxic.

There are some patients with muscle symptoms with normal CK, and the position here is less clear. In the randomised, double-blind clinical trials there are no significant numerical differences between placebo and active groups, although some patients were excluded in the run-in phase. Muscle symptoms more likely to be linked to the statin are those where there is generalised muscle discomfort, tenderness, weakness or pain, rather like the 'first day or two of influenza'.

7.8 What safety monitoring should be undertaken?

Safety monitoring of statin therapy is mainly clinical. Patients should be warned of the possible adverse event, but also told that it is very rare, and that treatment benefits greatly outweigh the risks. The drug package inserts for patients are not very helpful in referring to muscle pain or discomfort, because they do not give an indication of how relatively rare the symptoms are. Patients need to be told that the symptoms are not those related to joints, are not local pain in a single muscle area such as after unusual activity, and are not calf or other muscle cramps. Patients should be warned to report at the time any generalised muscle discomfort, pain, tenderness or weakness over day(s), with or without systemic upset, and perhaps feeling rather like 'the first days of influenza'. In practice most such episodes will be viral and not drug related, but the CK should be measured at the time and if there is clinical concern the statin should be stopped for a day or so until the CK is available.

Routine measurement of CK in the absence of symptoms is unlikely to be helpful, and indeed because of the variable nature of CK levels with exercise may give rise to false alarms.

It is appropriate to check hepatic, renal and thyroid function before statin initiation. It is reasonable to recheck ALT at 1–3 months when the first post-treatment lipid profile is being measured. Transaminases may be checked once or twice in the first year, but if they are normal, the statin dose is quite low, and there are no other significant medical problems, repeated subsequent measurement is unlikely to be helpful. However, any co-therapies need to be considered for the possibility of an increased interaction risk.

In asymptomatic patients, if in a routine measurement, a rise in ALT up to three times, and in CK up to five or even 10 times the upper limit of normal can be acceptable.

7.9 How should myalgia be managed?

When patients present with myalgia, history taking should establish whether symptoms are localised or generalised, their severity, and their relationship in time to initiation or change in statin or dose or other medication. That the presentation is truly myalgic (and not for example calf cramp or joint related) should be confirmed.

Patients should have their CK measured at their presentation with myalgia and, depending on severity of symptoms, the statin may be temporarily stopped until the CK result is available.

Some patients may develop significant generalised muscle discomfort without CK abnormality, and this may limit or prevent statin therapy. Some such patients will develop symptoms on any statin at any dose, but some individuals will be asymptomatic on one but not another statin.

The modest number of patients unable to take statins should be considered for alternative treatments particularly when their cardiovascular risk is high. Bile acid sequestrants, fibrates, ezetimibe and nicotinic acid may all be options, together with dietary plant stanols or sterols (*see Qs 6.13–6.15*).

7.10 What action should be taken for raised transaminases?

Significant liver disease caused by statins is very rare. Ideally, patients should have had liver function checked as one of the exclusionary tests of a secondary dyslipidaemia, before a statin has been started. This then allows a clearer assessment of a finding of raised transaminases.

> When raised transaminases are found in a patient taking a statin, the test should be repeated, for often a repeat value has returned to normal. Other potential causes for the abnormality should be sought. Other drugs, gallstones or high alcohol intake may be responsible. Particularly in the overweight individual, in those with high triglycerides, and in those with features of the metabolic syndrome moderate abnormalities in liver enzymes (ALT and AST, but not alkaline phosphatase) may reflect hepatic fatty change – NAFLD. Abdominal ultrasound may support this diagnosis.
> It should be remembered that patients with dyslipidaemias are still at risk of other causes of liver disease, which should be excluded.

7.11 What drug interactions are seen with statins?

> Like many drugs, statins are largely metabolised in the liver through the cytochrome P450 system, and therefore interactions for statins may occur (*Table 7.1*).

The P450 system has a number of isoenzymes through which different drugs are handled. Of the statins, simvastatin, lovastatin, cerivastatin and atorvastatin are metabolised through the 3A4 isoenzyme, and have more potential for interaction with agents such as ciclosporin, the 'conazoles, erythromycin and protease inhibitors. In this 3A4 category grapefruit juice, especially in large quantities, can also influence drug (and the particular statin) metabolism, and has become a contraindication. Fluvastatin and pravastatin are metabolised through CYP 2C9 and have fewer potential interactions, and fluvastatin has been used in a major trial with ciclosporin without side effects (ALERT).[3] Rosuvastatin is largely excreted unchanged,

TABLE 7.1 The metabolism of various drugs through the human cytochrome P450 isoenzyme system

CYP3A4	CYP2D6	CYP2C19	CYP2C9
Amiodarone	Amitriptyline	Diazepam	Alprenolol
Amlodipine	Bufaralol	Ibubrufen	Diclofenac
Atorvastatin	Codeine	Mephenytoin	Fluvastatin
Cerivastatin	Debrisoquine	Methyl-	Pravastatin
Clarithromycin	Dextro-	phenobarbital	Hexobarbital
Cyclosporine A	methorphan	Omeprazol	N-desmethyl-
Diltiazem	Encainide	Proguanyl	diazepam
Erythromycin	Flecainide	Phenytoin	Tolbutamide
Ketoconazole	Imipramine		Warfarin
Itraconazole	Metoprolol		
Lovastatin	Mibefradil		
Mibefradil	Nortriptyline	[Rosuvastatin has 10% metabolism	
Midazolam	Perhexiline	through CYP2C9 and CYP2C19]	
Nefazodone	Perphenazine		
Nifedipine	Propafenone		
Protease inhibitors	Propranolol		
Quinidine	Sparteine		
Sildenafil	Thioridazine		
Simvastatin	Timolol		
Terbinafine			

Modified from Ballantyne et al.[2]

with only 10% metabolised through 2C9 and 2C19, but as with the other statins ciclosporin raises rosuvastatin levels several-fold. Limitations have been placed on high-dose rosuvastatin use.

Interactions such as those of statins with warfarin require the anticoagulant effect to be watched in the first days after treatment, and a moderate dose adjustment may be required, but thereafter treatment should be stable.[2]

7.12 Are all statins the same?

All statins have the same mode of action, reducing cholesterol synthesis through partial blockade of HMG-CoA reductase. Their effects in reducing cardiovascular disease risk are all mediated through the resulting fall in LDL-cholesterol, and effects are proportional to the fall in LDL-cholesterol achieved.

Efficacy of statins at their starting dose varies. At their starting dose, all the statins will reduce LDL-cholesterol by at least 25% or substantially more with some. For all, each doubling of a statin dose will achieve approximately a further 5–6% fall in LDL-cholesterol. In terms of potency on a mg-per-mg basis, LDL lowering increases by 5–6% moving from pravastatin or fluvastatin to simvastatin, by 5–6% from simvastatin to atorvastatin, and by around 9% from atorvastatin to rosuvastatin. The statins do, however, vary in several ways related to their pharmacology – half life, open or closed ring, fungal or synthetic, lipophilic or hydrophilic, degree of binding to HMG-CoA reductase, and the proportion of the dose that enters the systemic circulation.

While the mode of action in lowering LDL-cholesterol is the same for all statins, they also raise high density lipoprotein (HDL)-cholesterol by between 5 and 10%, perhaps slightly more with fluvastatin and rosuvastatin and perhaps rather less with higher doses of atorvastatin. How much this independently or additionally influences risk of cardiovascular disease is uncertain, for there are close relationships between reduced cardiovascular events and cholesterol or LDL-cholesterol reductions. Similarly, various other actions not immediately related to LDL lowering have been reported with different statins. These 'pleiotropic' effects may still be indirectly linked to lowering LDL-cholesterol, and how much (if at all) they influence cardiovascular outcomes is uncertain. For example, various inflammatory markers, cytokines and vasoactive substances are altered. Elevated levels of high-sensitivity C-reactive protein (CRP) are clearly associated with cardiovascular risk. CRP levels fall quite quickly with statin use. How much this is directly or indirectly linked to, or is independent of, LDL lowering is uncertain. In addition, inhibition of the cholesterol synthetic pathway by statins (at high doses) may modulate the levels of side pathways from this main path. Thus some products of farnesylation or geranylgeranylation may modify the expression of inflammatory markers and cytokines. Such effects may differ between statins, but there is as yet no long-term evidence in randomised controlled trials (RCTs) of benefit in actual CVD outcome.

Duration of action with statins with shorter half-lives (lovastatin, pravastatin, fluvastatin and perhaps simvastatin) means that the efficacy is slightly greater on LDL-cholesterol (perhaps up to 3%) when the drugs are given at night rather than in the morning. When fluvastatin is given in the extended release format, its absorption is much slower, leading to a more continuous hepatic exposure and removal, with very little drug reaching the systemic circulation, and allows an increase of around 4–5% efficacy in LDL lowering over the standard fluvastatin preparation. However, atorvastatin and especially rosuvastatin have much longer half-lives, and there is no major advantage over precise timing of drug administration.

7.13 Do all statins have the same risk of side effects?

 Clearly, the risk of side effects from statins may differ between different agents. It was the finding of increased muscle disease that led to the

TABLE 7.2 Adverse event rates for statins from October 1997 to December 2000

	Cerivastatin	Lovastatin	Fluvastatin	Pravastatin	Simvastatin	Atorvastatin
Rhabdomyolysis	88.7	1.2	0.6	1.4	3.6	1.2
Myopathy	6.5	4.2	0.6	1.2	1.6	0.5
Myositis	11.5	3.9	0.2	1.0	1.3	0.6
Myalgia	46.3	16.4	2.7	5.8	7.5	8.0

Adverse events reported per one million US prescriptions for each statin.
Data from the FDA AERS database and Public Citizen (www.fda.gov) and Ballantyne et al.[2]

TABLE 7.3 Number of prescriptions for statin use in the USA and the reported cases of fatal rhabdomyolysis

	Lovastatin	Pravastatin	Simvastatin	Fluvastatin	Atorvastatin	Cerivastatin	Total
Fatal rhabdomyolysis	19	3	14	0	6	31	3
Number of scripts dispensed ($\times 10^6$)	99	81	116	37	140	9.8	484
Report rate ($\times 10^6$ scripts)	0.19	0.04	0.12	0	0.04	3.16	0.15

Data from the FDA AERS database and Public Citizen (www.fda.gov) and Ballantyne et al.[2]

withdrawal of cerivastatin in August 2001[2] (www.fda.gov; *Tables 7.2 and 7.3*). The risk of severe myositis associated with rhabdomyolysis was 25–140-fold higher with cerivastatin than with other available statins, and death rates at least 20–50-fold higher.

The risk of myositis with cerivastatin increased as the drug dose was escalated and in a proportion of people was very markedly increased and related to concurrent use of gemfibrozil. Acute myositis is more likely in women, in those with a small body mass and those more elderly, and in those with other severe disease or taking other medications metabolised through the cytochrome P450 system. In sensible use with statins other than cerivastatin, the risk of rhabdomyolysis is unlikely to be greater than once per 50 000 patient-years of treatment. Many tens of millions of patient-years' exposure to the longer established statins has established the rarity of the severest form of myositis with rhabdomyolysis, and this is reassuring.

7.14 If adverse effects occur with one statin, is it worth switching to another?

 It is often worth choosing an alternative statin as some symptoms noted on treatment may have been non-specific.

The significant or potentially threatening side effects of statins are rare. In the RCTs of statins there have not been significant differences in the rates of withdrawal from treatment between active and placebo groups. Therefore, if with one statin there are non-specific or limited musculoskeletal (without major CPK rise) symptoms it is usually appropriate to give an alternative statin, beginning with a low dose.

An individual who has acute myositis with one statin will have a substantially higher risk of reacting against other statins.

It should be established if the myositis may have been linked to co-administration of (an)other drug(s) that may have interfered with statin clearance. This may depend on the catabolic pathway of the particular statin and other drugs, and interactions are more common if the catabolic pathways are shared (*see Table 7.1*). Thus fluvastatin and pravastatin are catabolised through the cytochrome P450 2C9 pathway, while many drugs including atorvastatin, lovastatin, simvastatin (and the withdrawn cerivastatin) are catabolised through the 3A4 path. Despite the potential interactions, greater with dose escalation, the frequency is low, for example across the whole dose range of atorvastatin.

In patients who, in relation to statin therapy, have exhibited a rise in CK to greater than five or especially 10 times the upper limit of normal, care should be taken with re-exposure to statins. In the highest CVD risk patients where therapy has been troublesome it may be appropriate to seek specialist advice.

Disturbances of liver transaminases are rare with statins. Liver function should be checked prior to initial statin prescription. Abnormal liver function may be due to prior liver disorder. In addition, in patients with insulin resistance, with central adiposity, with mixed lipaemia and hypertriglyceridaemia, there may be raised transaminases secondary to NAFLD and hepatic fatty infiltration. NAFLD is not a contraindication to statin (or fibrate) use, but biochemical monitoring of liver function on treatment is appropriate.

7.15 Is it best to treat to target or use the doses used in clinical trials?

It is now clear that the major determinant of successful outcome with lipid lowering is related to the degree of fall in cholesterol and especially in LDL-cholesterol, which can have been achieved by diet, lifestyle, bile acid sequestrants (resins), nicotinic acid, statins and ileal bypass, or by various combinations thereof. It is likely, therefore, that it is the degree of LDL lowering that is critical rather than how it is achieved. With pravastatin the large outcome trials have used 40 mg daily, with fluvastatin 40–80 mg, with simvastatin 20–40 mg (4S started with 20 mg and titrated to 40 mg in a third), and with atorvastatin 10–80 mg.

In clinical use and in companies' drug licence, advice is to begin with the lower doses and titrate up. With atorvastatin initiation can now be across the dose range depending on the anticipated patient need. The CHD guidelines for prevention in the UK have previously suggested a need to lower cholesterol by 25% and to less than 5 mmol/L, and LDL-cholesterol by 30% and to less than 3 mmol/L, *whichever is greater*. Trials have suggested that the greater the fall the better, but full evidence for this awaits the outcomes in the next year or two of two further trials of different statin doses (SEARCH and IDEAL). The PROVE-IT study[4] compared 40 mg of pravastatin with 80 mg of atorvastatin, and the additional 16% lowering of LDL-cholesterol expected (and achieved) with the latter was associated with a 16% extra fall in CVD events. The TNT study[5] compared 10 mg and 80 mg atorvastatin in 10 001 patients over 4.9 years to achieve mean LDL-cholesterol levels of 2.6 and 2.0 mmol/L, respectively. The lower LDL level was associated with absolute and relative risk reductions in major cardiovascular events of 2.2% and 22%, respectively.

Patients should be treated to achieve a large fall in lipid levels, aiming to reach target if possible, and with new evidence to levels lower than current guidelines. Current guidelines date back to before the outcomes of newer trials, and have recently been revised.[6,7] The new UK Joint British Societies' guidelines[8] recognise the need to reduce cholesterol to <4 mmol/L and LDL-cholesterol to <2 mmol/L, and these are now the target values for all patients requiring treatment.

7.16   What are the implications of a poor response to treatment?

A poor response to therapy has a number of implications. Perhaps the most important is that the patient's CHD and stroke risk is then not going to have been significantly reduced.

Statins have a very significant capability of reducing cholesterol, and on the starting dose of a statin an average fall in LDL-cholesterol by 30% (or substantially more with some statins) is expected. Individual patients will vary, however, but it would be unusual not to see a 15–20% LDL reduction. Some individuals have higher rates of cholesterol gut absorption, and then tend to respond less well to the statin; they will, however, tend then to have more marked responses to ezetimibe when added to their statin.

As always, when response to a treatment is poor one needs to consider concordance with treatment. Tachyphylaxis is not seen with statins. It is recognised that many patients do not continue longer term their chronic disease treatments, and here discussion and agreement about shared care objectives between doctor and patient are essential.

FIBRATES

7.17   How do fibrates work?

The mode of action of fibrates is now more clearly understood. Fibrates interact with nuclear receptors leading to altered gene transcription. The receptor is called peroxisome proliferator-activated receptor alpha (PPAR-α), fibrates having opposite effects to saturated fatty acids. There are also PPAR-γ receptors, activated by thiazolidinediones (the 'glitazones') that are insulin sensitisers, useful in treating some patients with type 2 diabetes.

Fibrates reduce hepatic secretion of VLDLs, and activate peripheral tissue lipoprotein lipase increasing triglyceride clearance. When triglyceride-rich lipoproteins (chylomicrons and VLDLs) are cleared more rapidly, their metabolism leads to higher HDL levels. Lower levels and more rapid clearance of triglyceride also prevent the formation in the blood stream of altered LDL molecules. When triglycerides are high, smaller more dense triglyceride-enriched LDLs are formed which are more atherogenic. Fibrates lead to improved LDL quality (*see* Q 7.18).

7.18   What are the indications for a fibrate?

Fibrates have their greater effects in reducing hypertriglyceridaemia and raising HDL-cholesterol in patients with mixed hyperlipidaemia, and have smaller effects on LDL-cholesterol levels. However, it is well recognised that patients with this mixed hyperlipidaemia have altered quality of LDL molecules. When triglycerides are high there is increased exchange of triglycerides from VLDLs with cholesterol ester from LDLs and HDLs. The triglyceride from the triglyceride-enriched LDL is removed by hepatic lipase, and the LDL shrinks in size, and is called small, dense LDL or LDL_3. When small dense LDLs are the predominant form of LDL, for a given amount of LDL-cholesterol there are greater numbers of LDL molecules if there is excess LDL_3, and these molecules are more atherogenic.

In the American NCEP ATP-III guidelines,[9] after statins have reduced LDL sufficiently, then attention should be given to features of the metabolic syndrome (*see* Q 4.3), and if present then a fibrate addition to treatment may be appropriate.

Currently, in most patients with mixed hyperlipidaemia the initial treatment will still be a statin aiming to get LDL to target below 2 (previously <3) mmol/L. Thereafter, when patients continue to show significant levels of hypertriglyceridaemia, especially with a low HDL-cholesterol, then addition of a fibrate is appropriate. Gemfibrozil would not now be used in conjunction with a statin because of the increased myositis risk. Fenofibrate is usually well tolerated with a statin (and for fenofibrate there is accumulating safety data[10]), but bezafibrate or ciprofibrate are alternatives.

In patients with severe hypertriglyceridaemia (*see Fig. 4.6 and* Q 4.12) there are additional risks of acute pancreatitis (when triglycerides are >10 and especially >20 mmol/L). Here fibrates may be the initial treatment of choice, and statins are not helpful.

In patients with low LDL levels but hypertriglyceridaemia and other risks, again fibrates may be first choice.

In familial dysbetalipoproteinaemia (remnant lipaemia; type III hyperlipidaemia; *see* Q 4.11), fibrates are the treatment of choice.

7.19 What are the side effects of fibrates?

Fibrates may share with statins the risk of myositis, at a fairly similar incidence when used alone. A combination of fibrate with statin increases the risk although it remains very small.

Gemfibrozil has a significantly higher risk of myositis than other fibrates and should not be used with a statin. It is rarely the fibrate of choice now, despite outcome evidence from the Helsinki Heart Study[11] and the VA-HIT study.[12] The gemfibrozil interactions with other agents metabolised through the cytochrome P450 3A4 system (*see Table 7.1*) are one of the reasons, but other biochemical pathways are also responsible for this gemfibrozil risk.

All fibrates may occasionally be associated with usually minor gastrointestinal symptoms.

7.20 Are all fibrates the same?

While the modes of action of the fibrates are essentially the same, there are some differences in the pattern and efficacy in the resulting lipid changes, and there are clear differences in the potential for side effects.

The main effects are in the lowering of triglycerides and raising of HDL-cholesterol. Depending on the initial triglyceride levels there may be some lowering of LDL-cholesterol. As the catabolism and clearance of triglyceride-rich lipoproteins is accelerated with fibrates, LDL-cholesterol may change little in some patients with the higher initial plasma triglycerides. Fenofibrate may have modestly better effects on LDL-cholesterol than some other fibrates.

The potential side effects of fibrates do vary. Gemfibrozil is more likely to show interactions with potential side effects with other drugs and in particular with statins. When cerivastatin was found to have substantially higher rates of myositis compared to other statins, and leading to cerivastatin's withdrawal, the concurrent use of gemfibrozil was common. The present approach is likely to be avoidance of gemfibrozil use especially with a statin or with other drugs metabolised through the cytochrome P450 3A4 system (*see Table 7.1*).

Fibrates other than gemfibrozil are better tolerated and interactions with statins and other drugs are fewer. A large cerivastatin–fenofibrate study in diabetes was in progress at the time of cerivastatin withdrawal and then halted, but interactions with this drug combination were limited.

OTHER PHARMACOLOGICAL TREATMENTS

7.21 How does ezetimibe work?

Ezetimibe has a new mode of action as the first drug to inhibit cholesterol absorption. This is at the level of the enterocyte, and ezetimibe led to the identification of a specific transport system controlling cholesterol passage across the gut cell. When less cholesterol is absorbed, the liver will then supplement hepatic cholesterol levels from other sources. This can be partly from an increase in hepatic cholesterol synthesis, but also by increasing cholesterol (as LDL-cholesterol) uptake from the blood. Reduced cholesterol availability in the liver leads to upregulation of hepatic LDL receptors, and a fall in blood LDL-cholesterol levels.

This lowering of plasma LDL-cholesterol by increased hepatic LDL uptake occurs whenever the liver has a cholesterol requirement. A reduced dietary intake of cholesterol will have this effect as will the use of the bile acid sequestrants (resins). The action of the resins is of course different from ezetimibe, as the resins bind cholesterol that is then lost in the faeces whereas ezetimibe inhibits transport across the enterocyte. Ezetimibe is well tolerated, is taken as a single fixed dose, and does not have the gastrointestinal side effects of resins.

Ezetimibe is used in a fixed daily single dose of 10 mg, and there are no advantages and no significantly increased effects on LDLs from exceeding this dose. Currently the ezetimibe prescribing information does not recommend co-prescribing of fibrates with ezetimibe but a co-use paper has shown no untoward effect.[13] However, there are some high risk patients in whom their lipid abnormalities are sufficiently severe related to their clinical problems that such co-prescribing is used. Specialist advice should be sought for these individual patients.

7.22 What is the role of ezetimibe?

Ezetimibe is indicated as a therapy in patients with significant hypercholesterolaemia. It produces a fall in LDL-cholesterol of around 18%. Ezetimibe is unlikely to be a first line drug to be used alone as the LDL lowering ability is more limited than that of a statin.

The LDL reduction is similar when ezetimibe is sole therapy after diet, or when added to other drug regimens. The fall in LDL is a little less when used in a patient already on a maximum statin dose. There is some variation in the responses of individuals, just as there is some variation in response to statins. In those individuals who inherently have a greater ability to absorb cholesterol the statins may be a little less effective and ezetimibe a little more so. As a result the combination of statin and ezetimibe may have a particular role to maximise LDL-cholesterol lowering.

> It can be suggested that ezetimibe should be used with the lowest dose of a statin, the combination giving an LDL-lowering effect similar to the highest dose of that statin. However, additional LDL-lowering will result when ezetimibe is added to any statin dose, and for some higher risk patients needing greater LDL reduction ezetimibe with full dose statin will be appropriate. The statins have been widely used and studied across the dose ranges in clinical use and long-term trials, while long-term trials for ezetimibe are awaited to confirm that there are the expected outcome benefits, and to establish long-term side effects and safety.
>
> Ezetimibe availability does not preclude the use of the bile acid sequestrants which can have greater LDL lowering ability, but which in fuller dose can have significant gastrointestinal side effects. Ezetimibe is important for those patients who may be intolerant of statins and/or resins.

7.23 What are the side effects of ezetimibe?

Ezetimibe has been very well tolerated in the initial trials leading to licensing, and in its subsequent clinical use. No specific side effects for the drug have been identified. The side effect pattern of the drug studies has been very clean, even in animal toxicology studies where the drug was given at much higher doses than required. Long-term follow-up information in clinical use is awaited.

7.24 What is the role of omega-3 fish oil capsules?

Omega-3 fish oils have two main clinical effects: they lower triglycerides, and they influence the blood clotting pathways to decrease thrombotic tendency. The benefits will be present if taken naturally in the diet as fish, particularly as oily fishes, or if taken as a concentrated dietary supplement.[14] Taken as fish in the diet has aesthetic or culinary benefit of course, but will also have reduced intake of other fats (such as saturated animal fat) that might have otherwise been taken at that meal.

Supplements can be obtained from health food stores, but omega-3 fish oils are available as prescribable drugs.

Benefits in reducing heart attack rates are suggested from studies such as Caerphilly[15] where individuals taking higher amounts of fish in the diet had less CHD, and also in the GISSI-Prevenzione trial of fish oil supplements.[16]

> As 'Omacor', fish oil supplements are licensed at a lower dose of 1–2 g daily to reduce CHD risk, and at the higher dose of up to 4 g daily to lower triglycerides.

7.25 What is the role of nicotinic acid?

Nicotinic acid is not just a vitamin (at low dose), but when given at a high, pharmacological dose has hypolipidaemic effects.

Nicotinic acid acts in adipose tissue to inhibit triglyceride breakdown, and reduce the release of non-esterified ('free') fatty acids (NEFA). NEFA are carried bound to albumin back to the liver if not taken up by other tissues for energy supply. If the NEFA influx to the liver is reduced, so then is reduced the hepatic synthesis of triglycerides. The secretion not only of VLDLs but also of LDLs can be reduced as a result. Nicotinic acid is therefore a treatment for patients with hypertriglyceridaemia or with mixed hyperlipidaemia.

Early Scandinavian studies and the nicotinic acid arm of the American Coronary Drug Project have shown benefit in reducing CHD rates.

7.26 Why is nicotinic acid not used more widely?

This relates to the potential side effects of this agent. Many patients experience gastrointestinal side effects and marked flushing as doses are built up to 1.5–3 g/day. Building up the dose slowly from low levels can significantly minimise side effects, and taking aspirin (even in low dose) can limit the flushing. Liver function tests can be disturbed, and glucose tolerance can deteriorate, perhaps with short-acting rather than slow-release preparations.

Nicotinic acid also raises HDL levels better than other lipid-active therapies.

Nicotinic acid preparations are therefore not a first line therapy, but have a role in higher risk patients with difficult-to-control dyslipidaemia.

Now available in many countries is a slow-release preparation of nicotinic acid, Niaspan. Again dose should be built up over 2–3 weeks to limit initial side effects, and this can be a useful addition to treatment in some patients.

7.27 What is the role of bile acid sequestrants?

Bile acid sequestrants (resins) are a very effective therapy in lowering LDL-cholesterol, and older studies such as the Lipid Research Clinics – Coronary Primary Prevention Trial (LRC-CPPT)[17,18] and the St Thomas' Atherosclerosis Regression Study (STARS)[19] have confirmed benefit in reducing CHD. These resins (colestyramine and colestipol) were the mainstay of treatment before statins became available. They continue to be a useful treatment to use alone or with other therapies. Using 20–30 g of a resin will lower LDL-cholesterol by 30% or more, and even smaller doses of 5–10 g/day will reduce LDL-cholesterol by 15% or so.

The resins work within the gut by binding bile acids secreted from the liver in the bile. Normally, greater than 90% of bile acids are reabsorbed and recycled, but this is reduced by resins. Hepatic bile acid synthesis from cholesterol as a precursor therefore increases, and hepatic cell surface LDL receptors are upregulated to replenish hepatic cholesterol. As a result of the increased LDL uptake the plasma LDL-cholesterol falls. This altered hepatic metabolism is therefore similar to that which occurs when the inhibitor of cholesterol transport at the level of the enterocyte, ezetimibe, is used (*see Q 7.21*).

7.28 Why are resins used so much less now?

The resins have significant gastrointestinal side effects – of nausea, bloating, indigestion, constipation – that can be very limiting in some patients. They are powders that need to be mixed with food or a good volume of fluid such as water or orange juice and are slow to become suspended in the solution.

Resins remain useful, when tolerated, in moderate or higher dose as an adjunct to statins and other therapies, especially in high risk individuals needing greater lowering of LDL as with familial hypercholesterolaemia. They are not appropriate in individuals with significant hypertriglyceridaemia.

7.29 What are the roles of metformin and the thiazolidinediones?

These agents are not primarily drugs for the treatment of hyperlipidaemia or dyslipidaemia, but are used in type 2 diabetes as insulin sensitisers.

However, there are some moderate benefits of the thiazolidinediones in improving lipid profiles, part of which will be related to improved diabetic control, and part may be more direct. It is the mixed hyperlipidaemia and the quality of LDL that may be improved, with a switch away from small dense LDLs towards the less atherogenic larger LDL particles.[20] Actual LDL-cholesterol concentrations may not change or may increase by small amounts. For the same degree of improvement in haemoglobin A1c (HbA1c) there may be some differences of moderate degree in lipid profiles between the current marketed glitazones – rosiglitazone and pioglitazone – tending to favour pioglitazone.[21]

Metformin has similar effects as an insulin sensitiser and again changes in lipid profiles are of the same pattern and approach the same magnitude as with the glitazones. Metformin should be the first agent for treatment of significant hyperglycaemia in overweight type 2 diabetes, with the glitazones as second line, hypolipidaemic effects being a bonus. However, statins and then fibrates are still the agents of first choice for drug management of dyslipidaemia, after diet and lifestyle changes.

7.30 When is combination therapy required?

Combination therapy for lipid management may be required in a number of circumstances, and particularly in individuals at high cardiovascular risk. The combination of medications likely to be most efficacious will depend on the particular hyperlipidaemia or dyslipidaemia.

Patients who have already experienced cardiovascular disease are at particular risk of further disease, and if initial treatment fails to bring their lipid levels to target then additional treatment may be required. Similarly, those individuals with familial hypercholesterolaemia are at particular risk and have particularly elevated LDL-cholesterol. A further group of patients who have high risk are those with mixed hyperlipidaemia, with both elevated LDL-cholesterol and hypertriglyceridaemia, but often with associated low HDL-cholesterol. This latter group often has insulin resistance and/or diabetes mellitus and impaired glucose tolerance.

A final group of patients, where lipid control may be particularly difficult, have severe hypertriglyceridaemia (*see Fig. 4.6*), giving rise to a high risk of pancreatitis.

Thus in patients primarily requiring LDL lowering ezetimibe, resins and at times fenofibrate will be combined with a statin. For mixed lipaemia fibrates and nicotinic acid may be used with a statin. Some of these more difficult-to-control patients may be referred to secondary care for initial advice or at times shared care.

7.31 Which drug combinations are preferred?

Combinations of lipid-lowering drugs appropriate for the management of dyslipidaemia will vary depending on the pattern of lipid abnormality.

HYPERCHOLESTEROLAEMIA AND HIGH LDL-CHOLESTEROL

For patients with hypercholesterolaemia and high LDL-cholesterol values the initial preferred treatment would be a statin. Good outcome data are also available for resins[14,15] and statin–resin combinations are very appropriate. Tolerance of resins can be relatively poor, and in future a combination of a statin with the new inhibitor of cholesterol absorption, ezetimibe (see Q 7.21), is likely to be the treatment of choice (although long-term outcome of ezetimibe is not yet available). One could use low dose statin with ezetimibe, but the LDL lowering effect will be no different from using a fuller statin dose alone, cost may be more, and compliance with two medicines is likely to be lower than with one. This may be partly corrected with the combination preparation ezetimibe–simvastatin, but a combination tablet with other statins will not be forthcoming. With high LDL-cholesterol patients, with high risk patients, and as LDL targets are now lower at <2 mmol/L, ezetimibe will be valuable with full(er) doses of statins.

HIGH CARDIOVASCULAR RISK AND MIXED HYPERLIPIDAEMIA

Where individuals at high cardiovascular risk have mixed hyperlipidaemia, it would be usual to lower LDL-cholesterol to target first, usually with a statin. Where there is residual hypertriglyceridaemia, and particularly when HDL-cholesterol is low, a fibrate would be an appropriate addition. Fenofibrate, or perhaps bezafibrate, would be the agent of choice, normally being well tolerated, but gemfibrozil should be avoided, particularly in combination with a statin. Individually both statins and fibrates have a very rare risk of acute myositis, the risk being a little higher in combination, and patient education about the rare symptoms is important. In type III hyperlipidaemia (remnant lipaemia) a statin may be added where a fibrate alone has been insufficient.

An alternative to add to statins in patients with inadequately corrected mixed dyslipidaemia would be nicotinic acid, as the slow-release preparation Niaspan. This will lower both triglycerides and LDL-cholesterol and help raise HDL-cholesterol.

In high risk individuals with satisfactory LDL-cholesterol levels but with residual hypertriglyceridaemia, fibrate use may be initial therapy. Again a nicotinic acid preparation and/or a concentrated omega-3 fish oil preparation can be added to the fibrate.

SEVERE HYPERTRIGLYCERIDAEMIA

In patients with severe hypertriglyceridaemia >10 mmol/L, and especially if >20 mmol/L, the risk of acute pancreatitis is high. Secondary causes (diabetes, excess alcohol, obesity) need attention, but multiple therapies with fibrate, concentrated fish oil, and perhaps nicotinic acid, may be helpful. In the very rare patients whose severe hypertriglyceridaemia is due to deficiency of lipoprotein lipase (LPL) or apolipoprotein-CII, the mainstay of treatment is a very restricted fat intake to less than 10% of total calories, compared to the usual low fat diet of <30% of calories. Such a very restrictive diet is exceedingly demanding, and fortunately these patients are rare. There is a possibility in the next 2–3 years of a gene replacement therapy for lipoprotein lipase deficiency (*see Ch. 12*).

Where multiple therapies are being used, and where agents are being used at higher dose, then patients need to be reminded about the potential, albeit quite rare, side effects. Combination therapies may often be commenced in secondary care, and patients may be referred from primary care for advice and/or shared care.

ALTERNATIVE TREATMENTS

7.32 What radical therapy is available?

In patients with the very rare homozygous familial hypercholesterolaemia (*see Q 4.6*) (1 per million prevalence) drug therapy will be inadequate. In severe heterozygous familial hypercholesterolaemia, especially in some younger individuals who have a very poor family history for premature vascular disease, drug therapy may again be inadequate. There will also be patients with early severe cardiovascular disease with other inherited lipaemias or polygenic predisposition in whom statin treatment may be inadequate or not tolerated, where alternative treatment will be required.

These individuals should be referred to specialist lipid–cardiovascular disease secondary care centres. Here they can be considered for LDL-apheresis, and referred on to the small number of tertiary centres where this may be available. Currently access to LDL-apheresis is inappropriately limited, but should gradually become more readily available.

LDL-apheresis involves attachment of the patient to a machine through which plasma or whole blood is run through columns that will remove LDL-cholesterol. Related to the synthetic rate of LDL, the process has to be carried out fortnightly. Specialist centres provide LDL-apheresis, but this is more likely to be carried out in renal dialysis or blood transfusion centres. From a patient point of view the process is rather akin to renal dialysis procedures.

In the next few years we are likely to see new drug groups developing. Perhaps further agents will selectively modulate the PPAR system with more lipid-specific actions maximising the beneficial effects of fibrates with thiazolidinediones without the adipogenic stimulus. Development of partial inhibitors of cholesterol ester transfer protein (CETP) are likely to allow a major increase in HDL-cholesterol levels and markedly improve LDL quality.

For the very rare individual with inherited deficiency of lipoprotein lipase (approximately 1 per million population) and who has suffered (and often recurrently) acute pancreatitis, it is possible that gene replacement therapy for lipoprotein lipase will become available over the next few years.

PATIENT QUESTIONS

7.33 What alternative therapies are available for raised cholesterol and blood fats?

The first management for abnormal blood fats should be attention to lifestyle. In different individuals attention to diet, alcohol, weight, exercise and fitness are variably important. Drug therapy should be added to these measures; drugs should not be a substitute.

The alternative drug therapies for abnormal blood fats fall into different groups. Some drugs are best at lowering blood cholesterol, others are better at lowering blood triglyceride fat, and others may affect both cholesterol and triglyceride. The treatments that are best at lowering cholesterol (and the 'bad' LDL-cholesterol) are statins, bile acid sequestrants (resins) and ezetimibe. Where high blood triglycerides are the main problem, fibrates, fish oils and nicotinic acid are the agents best suited. Some people will need combinations of therapy.

For many patients who already have heart disease or have suffered a stroke, drug therapy will be essential. Individuals with inherited disorders of cholesterol and nearly all with diabetes will also need treatment. For people at lower risk the diet and lifestyle changes may be sufficient without adding drugs. In everyone moderate further benefits in lowering LDL-cholesterol (by perhaps 10% on average) can be achieved by taking sufficient food spreads or other foods containing plant stanols and sterols (Benecol and Flora-Proactive).

Concentrated fish oils in high dose can lower triglycerides. In more moderate dose the fish oils can limit blood clotting, and through this can limit thrombosis risk.

Alternative medicine and health stores have a wide range of possible treatments that are said to reduce lipids and vascular risk, but few of these have any firm evidence of benefit. They may not have evidence of harm, but harm may be done if these are taken instead of proven remedies.

7.34 Do drugs cure the problem?

Drug therapies do not 'cure' the problem of either abnormal blood fats, or the risk for first or further vascular disease events. Diet and lifestyle measures, and drug therapies, reduce the future risk – often quite substantially – but do not remove all risk.

Risk needs to be assessed in all individuals. Clearly a person who has already had a circulatory problem (such as stroke, angina or heart attack) has a much higher risk of a further problem than someone who has been healthy. If one considers the next year or the next decade, older people have a much higher risk than younger. However, if a risk factor is elevated in the young then their lifetime risk is much greater than when an abnormal risk factor first develops in an older person.

Treatments need to be targeted at those individuals with high risk. While no individual is immune from vascular risk, drug therapy should not be targeted to the very low risk end of the population. Available now is low dose statin treatment from the pharmacist (subject to fulfilling a risk assessment algorithm) to certain moderate risk individuals who have not yet experienced a clinical event.

If a person has sufficient risk of heart disease or stroke then treatment should be targeted not just to one but to all the risk factors that are present that contribute to this increased risk. One cannot alter gender, age or family history, but blood cholesterol and triglyceride fats, high blood pressure and smoking can be altered, and control of blood sugar levels in diabetes improved.

When drug treatments are needed for cholesterol, blood fats, blood pressure or diabetes these are lifelong and not short-lived treatments.

7.35 At what time of day should lipid-lowering medication be taken?

Statin and fibrate drugs are classically given at night. The reason for this is that the LDL-cholesterol lowering effect is a little greater than when the drug is given in the morning. However, when occasionally a combination of statin and fibrate is given, it is usual to take one at night (the statin) and one in the morning. With longer acting-statins (e.g. atorvastatin and rosuvastatin) there is no significant advantage in giving the drug at any particular time as the duration of action of the drug lasts throughout the 24 hours.

Ezetimibe is a once-daily preparation, and change of time of taking has little effect.

Different considerations apply to some of the other lipid lowering agents. The bile acid sequestrants (resins) are better tolerated and more effective when the dose is split through the day, and usually better not taken on an empty stomach. One of the problems with resin therapy is that absorption of other drugs that may be needed can be impaired. As a result it is advisable to take any other needed drugs 1 hour prior to, or 3–4 hours after, the resin which can be a significant inconvenience.

Nicotinic acid is best commenced at low dose and built up over a few weeks. It is better tolerated if taken with food two or three times daily.

7.36 Do lipid-lowering drugs cause impotence?

There is no evidence that lipid-lowering drugs cause impotence. Unfortunately, the underlying narrowing of the main arteries that causes heart disease and stroke can also affect the arteries to the abdomen and penis. As a result impotence may be part of the underlying artery disease rather than the cholesterol-lowering drugs that may be being taken.

7.37 How do I know if lipid-lowering drugs are being effective?

It is now recognised that what determines the effectiveness of treatment is how well treatment has lowered the blood cholesterol, or the blood level of the 'bad' cholesterol – the LDL-cholesterol – rather than the specific treatment or drug being used. However, there are also major research studies that have shown how effective diet and lifestyle changes, and drug treatments, are in lowering cholesterol. Of these, the trials with statin drugs have been the most extensive and the most effective. Monitoring the blood cholesterol (or LDL-cholesterol) is therefore the best way to monitor the likely effectiveness of lifestyle, diet and drug treatments.

There are additional beneficial effects likely to be gained from lowering high blood triglycerides or raising low HDL-cholesterol levels, which may occur with fibrates, nicotinic acid or fish oils. These can be monitored when a fasting lipid profile is measured.

The degree of coronary artery narrowing is assessed by an individual's exercise ability. Symptoms in daily life are one measure, but this can be formalised in a graded exercise test on a treadmill. This is not normally carried out routinely – only if there are concerns of an inadequate ability. More direct assessment of the arteries can be achieved by the X-ray test of coronary arteriography, where dye is injected to outline the arteries. This does have a small degree of risk, and is primarily carried out where it is likely that the patient will need treatment to the coronary arteries.

Various other tests can give additional information such as ultrasound examinations of heart muscle movement and efficiency, radioactive isotope studies of heart muscle function, scans to measure how much calcification ('chalk') there is in the arteries, and (as a research tool) ultrasound examination of the thickness of the arteries. This last test (called intravascular ultrasound) is performed by putting a probe inside each of the arteries to be examined; it is not without some risk, and clearly is not a routine investigation.

7.38 What other drugs are advised in patients at high cardiovascular risk?

Patients at high cardiovascular risk may not only need lipid-lowering treatment, but also other treatments. High blood pressure will need to be lowered. Aspirin in low dose protects against first or later heart attack or stroke and should be taken once any high blood pressure has been controlled. In some circumstances the anticoagulant warfarin may be used, and the anti-platelet drug clopidogrel may be used instead of low dose aspirin.

In patients who have had a heart attack, a beta-blocker (such as atenolol) has benefits partly protecting against a further attack. Drugs called angiotensin-converting enzyme inhibitors (or alternatively a related drug group, the angiotensin-receptor blockers) can be beneficial and protective, particularly if there has been any previous heart failure.

Individuals with diabetes will need to take treatment to control their blood sugar levels as much as possible, as this will reduce their risk. Treatments to help reduce weight (e.g. orlistat) can also be of benefit by tending to improve cholesterol and triglycerides, lower blood pressure, control blood sugar and even prevent or delay the onset of diabetes in persons at risk. It had been thought that treating the diabetes for up to 3–12 months after a heart attack with insulin (rather than diet, or diet and pills) was beneficial, but recent studies have not fully confirmed this. Nonetheless, one would wish to have good diabetic control achieved by any of the treatment options.

Drug treatment – clinical trial evidence

8.1	What was the experience of the early clinical trials?	130
8.2	What was the impact of the Scandinavian Simvastatin Survival Study?	130
8.3	What contribution did CARE, LIPID and other statin studies make to the secondary prevention of cardiovascular disease?	131
8.4	What did WOSCOPS, AFCAPS/TexCAPS, ASCOT-LLA and CARDS contribute to the primary prevention of cardiovascular disease?	132
8.5	How did the Heart Protection Study extend the evidence base further?	133
8.6	What contribution have recent trials made to the evidence base?	134
8.7	What outcomes are expected from current ongoing trials?	134

PQ PATIENT QUESTIONS

8.8	Do clinical trials reflect the real world?	136
8.9	Would every adult benefit from a statin?	137

8.1 What was the experience of the early clinical trials?

A number of early studies suggested benefits in reducing blood lipids and reducing coronary disease. However, many of these studies were of too small size, in lower risk populations, and used less effective or less well tolerated drugs. At this time there was a greater belief that it would be possible to prevent disease in individuals who had not yet had a clinical event, and less belief that it might be possible to prevent recurrent events. Studies were often not of sufficient size to be powered to examine reductions in total mortality and were able to look only at coronary events.

None the less, there were studies showing benefits from diet and lifestyle change, from nicotinic acid, from gemfibrozil and from bile acid sequestrants (resins). Important studies included, for example:

- the Helsinki Heart Study (HHS) with gemfibrozil[1]
- the Lipid Research Clinics – Coronary Primary Prevention Trial (LRC-CPPT) with colestyramine[2,3]
- the St Thomas' Hospital Atherosclerosis Regression Study (STARS) with diet, and with colestyramine.[4]

Meta-analyses of these and other studies confirmed the benefits of cholesterol lowering, suggesting that a 1% fall in low density lipoprotein (LDL)-cholesterol was associated with a 2% reduction in coronary risk. That lowering cholesterol caused violence or suicide (in LRC-CPPT and HHS studies) was refuted by the USA Food and Drug Administration.

From the 14-year observational study of 356 000 male screenees in the Multiple Risk Factor Intervention Trial (MRFIT),[5] any apparent excess of mortality from cancer in those with a low initial cholesterol was limited to the first year or two, and not later. This was due to a number of people entering the observation with existing malignancy (often bowel) or developing malignancy in that first year. Thus the catabolic effect of a malignancy was lowering the cholesterol, rather than the low cholesterol having any role in the disease development.

8.2 What was the impact of the Scandinavian Simvastatin Survival Study?

The Scandinavian Simvastatin Survival Study (4S), published in 1994,[6] was a pivotal study that changed international beliefs and practice. Over a period of 5.4 years the study investigators examined 4444 Scandinavian men and women (20%) with coronary heart disease (CHD), aged 35–70 years, with initial cholesterol values of 5.5–8.0 mmol/L. Patients were allocated to simvastatin or placebo. Initially active treatment was 20 mg simvastatin daily, but patients were then titrated either down to 10 mg (only two patients) or up to 40 mg so that the modal dose was 27 mg daily. Coronary mortality, coronary events, revascularisations and total mortality were reduced by 42, 34, 37 and 30%, respectively, but there were no significant differences in adverse events or withdrawal rates between the verum and placebo groups.

This study demonstrated that to treat individuals with heart attacks or CHD was not to 'shut the stable door after the horse had bolted'. In the decade since these results were published it has become routine for cardiologists and physicians to consider that all patients with CHD should be treated with a statin. It is recognised that this intention does not always reach fruition, and that there is still a significant treatment gap. It also showed that the small subgroup of patients with diabetes benefited at least as much if not more, and these data were later extended when the revised criteria from the American Diabetes Association for the diagnosis of diabetes and impaired fasting glycaemia were applied.[7]

Subsequent studies have extended the information obtained from the 4S study. Patients in subsequent prevention trials (some secondary and some primary) have had lower initial cholesterol levels, wider age ranges, included more females, and involved those with additional diseases such as hypertension and diabetes. A wide range of cardiovascular events have been prevented, importantly including stroke.

8.3 What contribution did CARE, LIPID and other statin studies make to the secondary prevention of cardiovascular disease?

CARE in the USA,[8] and LIPID mainly in Australia,[9] were two further secondary prevention trials that reported subsequent to the 4S trial. They confirmed that statin therapy was beneficial in secondary prevention of CHD and extended the evidence base. They included patients at lower overall risk and with lower initial cholesterol levels of 3.3–6 and 4–7 mmol/L, respectively, and extended the benefits to pravastatin (in a dose of 40 mg daily). Over 5 years the overall relative risk reduction in CARE was 24% in 4159 patients aged 21–75 years with a mean LDL-cholesterol of 3.59 mmol/L. In LIPID, 9014 patients aged 31–75 years with a mean LDL-cholesterol of 3.8 mmol/L were studied over 6.1 years with significant reductions of 24% in coronary and 22% in total mortalities. Subgroup analyses confirmed that there were few if any differences for those with hypertension, with diabetes,[10] who smoked or had had prior revascularisations, compared to those without these factors.

The LIPS study[11] showed reduction of risk with fluvastatin in patients recently undergoing angioplasty, while the ALERT study[12] showed benefit and safety of fluvastatin in renal transplant individuals receiving ciclosporin.

8.4 What did WOSCOPS, AFCAPS/TexCAPS, ASCOT-LLA and CARDS contribute to the primary prevention of cardiovascular disease?

WOSCOPS

The second major statin randomised controlled trial to report, and the first for primary prevention, was the West of Scotland Coronary Prevention Study (WOSCOPS).[13] This used 40 mg pravastatin daily in 6595 males (average age 60 years) with a mean LDL-cholesterol of 4.97 mmol/L. There was a 31% reduction in the primary endpoint of coronary events and deaths. The study was not powered to look at change in total mortality, but this was of borderline significant reduction at $p = 0.051$.

AFCAPS/TEXCAPS

In the Air Force Coronary Artery Prevention Study/Texas University Coronary Artery Prevention Study (AFCAPS/TexCAPS) 6605 males and females aged 45–73 years who had no history of CHD were studied over 5.2 years.[14] These patients were chosen to have an 'average' LDL-cholesterol (mean 3.89 mmol/L) but a low high density lipoprotein (HDL)-cholesterol (mean 0.94 mmol/L) and received 20 mg lovastatin, titrated to 40 mg daily, with the intent to reach a target LDL-cholesterol <2.9 mmol/L. They achieved a 37% (p <0.001) fall in the primary endpoint of combined fatal and non-fatal myocardial infarction, sudden death and unstable angina.

AFCAPS/TexCAPS showed significant benefits at least as good as, if not better than, those in other statin studies, but in a primary prevention group with the lowest absolute CHD risk (~6%/10 years) of the statin studies to date. It suggested that statins to lower LDL-cholesterol were valuable in individuals with low HDL-cholesterol, and provided evidence for a third statin, lovastatin.

ASCOT-LLA

The Lipid-Lowering Arm of the Anglo-Scandinavian Cardiac Outcomes Trial (ASCOT-LLA)[15] looked at over 10 000 patients (about half of the 19 500 patients in the main hypertension treatment study) given either 10 mg atorvastatin or placebo. Because these patients had such successful treatment of their hypertension, the CHD rate in the placebo group was only 9%/10 years. Nonetheless, rates of CHD and stroke were reduced by 36% and 27%, respectively.

Safe and effective reduction of cardiovascular disease (CVD) risk has therefore been seen in patients at low CVD risk in both ASCOT-LLA and AFCAPS/TexCAPS.

CARDS

The Collaborative Atorvastatin Diabetes Study (CARDS)[16] investigated primary prevention of vascular disease by the administration of 10 mg atorvastatin daily in 2838 patients with type 2 diabetes. This was the first study involving solely type 2 diabetics, and complements the Heart Protection Study (HPS) diabetes subset. This study terminated 2 years early because of a clear benefit in the treated group compared to the placebo group. A difference of 1.2 mmol/L in LDL-cholesterol was achieved between the two groups, leading to a 37% reduction in cardiovascular deaths and events. A 48% fall in strokes was seen. Some patients in the active treatment group ceased their statin (approximately 15%) and some placebo patients (9%) took a non-study statin. This dilutes out the apparent benefit, for taking atorvastatin 10 mg daily rather than not would reduce cardiovascular events by 49% and stroke by 64%. The number need to treat (NNT) to prevent one event over 5 years is 22. Reduction of total mortality on an intention to treat basis was 25%, but because the trial was prematurely terminated with fewer (by one-third) events than would otherwise have occurred, this did not reach statistical significance ($p = 0.059$).

8.5 How did the Heart Protection Study extend the evidence base further?

The Heart Protection Study (HPS)[17] was the largest study undertaken and had two components:

- ◼ simvastation 40 mg daily vs. placebo
- ◼ in a 2 × 2 factorial design, it examined an anti-oxidant vitamin mixture of vitamin C, vitamin E and beta-carotene.

There were 20 536 high risk individuals, two-thirds with existing vascular disease and one-third with diabetes or hypertension. Patients were aged 40–80 years (half >65 years) and the only lipid entry criterion was a cholesterol >3.5 mmol/L.

The anti-oxidant vitamins showed absolutely no difference between the active and placebo groups in either cardiac outcomes or in side effects.

In the statin part of the study, patients received simvastatin 40 mg daily or placebo. A reduction in LDL-cholesterol of approximately 1.0 mmol/L was achieved. All-cause and cardiac mortalities were reduced by 13 and 17%, respectively. Coronary events, revascularisations and strokes were reduced by 27, 24 and 25%, respectively. By Year 5 of the study, 18% of the active group were not taking their statin, but a third of the placebo group were taking a non-study statin, effectively diluting study outcomes by 50%. The achieved outcomes on an intention to treat basis of 27, 24 and 25% would therefore be augmented to 40, 36 and 37%, respectively.

HPS was large enough to have the power to examine subgroups prospectively. The nearly 6000 patients with diabetes showed clear and equal benefit compared to those without diabetes, and the 25% of females showed similar relative risk reductions to the males.[18] Those aged >75 years had similar relative risk reductions (at a higher absolute risk) than younger patients. The demonstrated stroke reduction was an intended prospective analysis.

There was no evidence of heterogeneity amongst all the subgroups selected, suggesting that the outcomes apply to all these subgroups.

8.6   What contribution have recent trials made to the evidence base?

From the recent statin studies it is clear that lowering cholesterol, and specifically LDL-cholesterol, substantially reduces CHD and stroke. A fall in LDL-cholesterol of about 1 mmol/L is associated with about a one-third reduction in cardiovascular risk, irrespective of the statin used in the trials. Including the older studies other than those with statins suggests that it is the LDL lowering that is important rather than how it is achieved. Studies with greater LDL lowering have achieved greater percentage event reduction.

A major contribution from the recent trials has been to demonstrate prospectively major reductions in stroke risk at least as good as for CHD reduction, despite a much flatter epidemiological relationship between stroke risk and cholesterol. Prevented strokes also make a substantial positive contribution to health economic outcomes.

Benefit is seen in all the groups studied: in primary and secondary prevention, in males and females, at all ages, across a wide range of cholesterol and LDL-cholesterol levels, and with or without other factors such as diabetes, hypertension or tobacco use. They have also demonstrated benefit down to cholesterol and LDL-cholesterol levels well below 4 and 2 mmol/L, respectively.

8.7   What outcomes are expected from current ongoing trials?

Within the next year or so we should see the results of further studies looking at patients randomised to two different statin doses:

- simvastatin 20:80 mg daily (the SEARCH trial)
- simvastatin 20 mg:atorvastatin 80 mg (the IDEAL study)
- fenofibrate and placebo (the FIELD study)

These should confirm the view that the lower the LDL-cholesterol achieved the better.

That this is likely is further suggested by the result of the PROVE-IT study[19] where the effects of pravastatin 40 mg daily were compared to atorvastatin 80 mg daily. This study is of particular interest as it was funded and run by the pravastatin manufacturers. They had believed that pravastatin had beneficial actions on atheroma outside lipid lowering not shown by the other statins. They also believed that there was an LDL threshold below which there was no further benefit of lipid lowering. The aim of the study had been to show non-inferiority of pravastatin compared to atorvastatin. These beliefs were proved unfounded. A difference of about 16% in LDL-cholesterol achieved (2.5 mmol/L:1.6 mmol/L) was associated with a further 16% reduction in CHD in the atorvastatin group. This study suggests an even lower LDL-cholesterol target may be appropriate and to be safe. Similarly, the TNT study[20] showed a 22% reduction in CVD risk when LDL was lowered to 2.0 mmol/L on 80 mg atorvastatin, compared to 2.6 mmol/L on 10 mg atorvastatin (see Q 7.15). There is now extensive evidence to suggest that there is no current lower threshold for LDL-cholesterol levels. In substantial numbers of patients LDL-cholesterol levels have been reduced to <1.5–2.0 mmol/L, with benefit, in HPS, ASCOT-LLA, CARDS, GREACE, LIPS, ALERT, PROVE-IT and TNT.

Levels of LDL-cholesterol are very low in the first year of life. LDL-cholesterol levels are substantially lower in Asian populations than in westernised populations,[21] and carry a much lower CHD risk. When Japanese populations move from Japan to Hawaii and California and take up the lifestyle of those areas, both cholesterol levels and coronary risk increase.

These findings have influenced the development of the new Joint British Societies' guidelines[22] for the primary prevention of cardiovascular disease with targets for high-risk patients of a cholesterol of <4 mmol/L and an LDL-cholesterol of <2 mmol/L. They have also led to a further report in the USA adjusting the guidelines from the National Cholesterol Education Program Adult Treatment Panel Third Report (NCEP ATP-III)[23] from LDL targets of <100 mg/dL (2.6 mmol/L) for high risk and <130 mg/dL (3.4 mmol/L) for moderately high-risk patients to lower values of <70 mg/dL (1.8 mmol/L) and <100 mg/dL (2.6 mmol/L), respectively.

Some uncertainty still exists in respect of the value of lowering of blood triglyceride levels independent of LDL-cholesterol, although lowering triglycerides in patients with lower HDL-cholesterol levels appears to have benefit. In the next year the results of the Fenofibrate Intervention and Event Lowering in Diabetes (FIELD) study should show whether there is benefit of fenofibrate compared to placebo in patients with diabetes. These patients were aged 50–70 years with a diabetes onset at age 35 years or greater, and were at risk of CHD without clear indication or contraindication for cholesterol lowering. The lipid criteria were baseline cholesterol of 3.0–6.5 mmol/L, together with a cholesterol/HDL ratio ≥4.0 or triglycerides >1.0 mmol/L. The USA guidelines (NCEP-ATPIII)[22] consider the metabolic syndrome (*see* Q 4.3) to be a secondary target for treatment after LDL-cholesterol, and the dyslipidaemia in these patients is likely to include raised triglycerides and low HDL-cholesterol, and to be suitable for fibrate treatment.

PATIENT QUESTIONS

8.8 Do clinical trials reflect the real world?

Clinical trials can provide reliable methods for assessing the efficacy of a treatment either against no treatment, or against the current best available treatment. The method of carrying out the trial, its length and its size are important if the relevant questions being asked are to be answered satisfactorily.

The trials of lowering cholesterol and blood fat have been among the biggest, longest and best designed of studies in any condition. These trials are designed as randomised controlled trials (RCTs), where patients are randomly allocated in a blinded manner to active or placebo treatment; there should therefore be no differences between the two groups to cause significant bias, particularly in these very large trials.

However, the studies do have limitations. There are rules called inclusion and exclusion criteria determining who is entered into the trials, and these effectively limit the applicability of the study concerned to a limited subset of the general population. Furthermore, not all eligible patients will agree to take part in a research study. It is recognised that patients not entering a trial are likely to have some differences (usually making them more at risk) from those included in the trial.

As there have been many statin trials with different agents and with different inclusion criteria, the results are likely to apply fairly well to the general population as similar results have been seen in all the trials and across all the patient subgroups.

Within trials some patients do move out from their allotted group and allotted treatment. Some patients may stop their allotted statin (drop-out) and some patients on placebo may be given a statin from outside the trial (drop-in). Such drop-outs and drop-ins reduce the power of a research trial, and mean that when a statin is taken 'in the real world' the benefit should be greater than seen in the trials.

A huge problem 'in the real world' is that many people cease their long-term medication, or take it intermittently or irregularly. To achieve the benefits seen in clinical trials does of course require the medication to be taken regularly.

8.9   Would every adult benefit from a statin?

Any adult at significant risk of a macrovascular event (coronary heart disease or stroke) will benefit from a statin if they have average or raised cholesterol or LDL-cholesterol levels. Benefits are evident down to LDL-cholesterol levels substantially below the levels in the great majority of the population. But what is a 'significant risk' in this respect?

- Individuals who have clinical vascular disease are at very high risk, as are patients with severe inherited hyperlipidaemias.
- Nearly all adults with diabetes have a significant risk.
- Individuals in whom the combination of their risk factors places them at ≥20%/10 year CVD risk.

It is the evidence from the AFCAPS/TexCAPS and ASCOT-LLA studies in particular and the safety of statins in general that have created a change in statin availability in the UK, which may be followed later in other countries. Now a generic preparation following the expiry of patent, simvastatin is currently available at the low 10 mg daily dose as a pharmacist-controlled preparation to lower/moderate risk individuals, i.e. males ≥55 years of age, or with one other risk factor (tobacco use, obesity, family history of premature cardiovascular disease, Asian), in males ≥45 years and females ≥55 years, where coronary heart disease risk is likely to be 8–15%/10 years and cardiovascular disease (with stroke) risk is likely to be 10–20%. These are individuals who will have a 1 in 10 to a 1 in 7 coronary heart disease risk over 10 years. Because a large number of individuals will need to take a drug over a significant period of years for only a moderate number to have avoided a cardiovascular event or death, there must be clear personal choice in this matter.

Individuals below these risk rates should not be taking statin therapy.

Implementing best practice

9.1	What is the extent of undertreatment?	140
9.2	What are the obstacles to effective implementation?	140
9.3	How is best practice implemented?	141
9.4	What guidelines are available to inform best practice?	141
9.5	What are the target lipid levels?	141
9.6	What are the pros and cons of targets?	142
9.7	Is total cholesterol the best target?	144
9.8	What is non-HDL-cholesterol?	147
9.9	Are target levels attainable?	147
9.10	What are the strategies to achieve target lipid levels?	148
9.11	How often should lipids be checked once at target?	148
9.12	How important is global risk factor modification?	148
9.13	How common is poor compliance?	149
9.14	What can be done to improve compliance?	150
9.15	Who should be referred to a specialist lipid clinic?	150
9.16	Why have statins been made available 'over the counter'?	151
9.17	What are the concerns surrounding 'over-the-counter' statins?	152

PQ PATIENT QUESTION
9.18 Who should take 'over-the-counter' statins?	153

9.1   What is the extent of undertreatment?

> Despite the compelling evidence of the clinical trials and widespread endorsement of lipid modification in individuals at risk, there remains a wide therapeutic gap between consensus recommendations and their implementation.

The large European survey, EUROASPIRE 2, showed that only 63% of a secondary prevention cohort was receiving lipid-lowering medication and 59% of patients still had cholesterol levels higher than 5.0 mmol/L.[1] A large survey of 2.4 million patients in 24 localities in England identified 89 422 patients with coronary heart disease (CHD).[2] Of the 78 600 whose records could be electronically interrogated by the data extraction tool MIQUEST, only 48% had a recording of total cholesterol. Of these, only 55% were receiving a statin and only 53% of these patients achieved target cholesterol levels of <5.0 mmol/L. The 'rule of halves', so commonly demonstrated in the management of hypertension, seems to be active in the management of hyperlipidaemia.

An equally gloomy picture is seen in the USA where Pearson et al found in the Lipid Treatment Assessment Project that, among 4888 patients, only 38% achieved target National Cholesterol Education Program (NCEP) low density lipoprotein (LDL) cholesterol goals and that of 1460 CHD patients, only 18% achieved the LDL-cholesterol goal of <100 mg/dL (<2.6 mmol/L).[3]

9.2   What are the obstacles to effective implementation?

Health professionals differ in their knowledge base, beliefs and the perception of their role in cardiovascular disease prevention. Cardiovascular disease prevention is a major undertaking to achieve systematically across the range of risk factors, and busy health professionals, beset by a demand-led service, are often concerned about their existing workload and resistant to change.

Implementation of long-term strategies is a role for primary care but practitioners may still be influenced by past controversies, concerned about adverse effects, or naturally nihilistic and conservative. For many, budgetary constraints are important but politically expedient decisions to limit expenditure may prove more expensive in the longer term. Current resource constraints mean that many practitioners lack the infrastructure – in terms of ancillary personnel, information technology and models of care – to provide appropriate support and follow-up.

Support for health professionals themselves should include appropriate education and training in the identification and management of patients. Patients chosen for treatment often reveal selection bias, and age, gender, race, weight, educational attainment, socio-economic status, geographic region and physician specialty have all been shown to strongly influence lipid management decisions.

Barriers to the implementation of cardiovascular disease prevention strategies also arise within patients. Patients tend to overestimate their health and the influences of family members, friends, the media and even different health professionals, all of which affect the knowledge, fears and perceptions that each individual brings with them.

9.3   How is best practice implemented?

The directing principles of best practice are set down in consensus guidelines or blueprints that health professionals can use for the management of groups and individuals at cardiovascular risk. To be effective, guidelines should be simple, consistent, evidence-based, achievable and cost-effective. Their uptake is enhanced if they reflect local needs and priorities, if they are multidisciplinary and if local agreement develops the feeling of ownership.

Multidisciplinary activity is important where the number of people to be managed is high and in cardiovascular disease prevention other health professionals, particularly nurses, are integral to successful programmes. The extended role of nurses has been examined in a randomised trial from north-east Scotland where improvements in drug prescription and risk factor modification after 1 year, in a CHD secondary prevention population, translated, after 4.7 years, into a significant 25% reduction in the death rate.[4]

The success of any clinical management programme is enhanced by audit. The development of robust audit systems which are computer-based and ongoing is an integral part of the governance structure that must be built into modern clinical management systems.

Financial reward is probably the most potent incentive to encourage the implementation of best practice and this is recognised in the new General Medical Services (GMS) contract for GPs in the UK where payments are made for the attainment of various quality standards (*see* Q *9.10*). With regard to lipid management, this will involve the secondary prevention of CHD and stroke and the management of diabetes.

9.4   What guidelines are available to inform best practice?

Guidelines for best practice from the UK, Europe and the USA are outlined in *Box 9.1*.

9.5   What are the target lipid levels?

Although consensus guidelines recommend target lipid levels (*Table 9.1*), the precise goals of therapy remain unknown. Recent clinical trials such as HPS, LIPS, ASCOT and CARDS suggest benefit when even lower levels of

> **BOX 9.1 Guidelines for best practice from the UK, Europe and the USA**
>
> **UK**
> - British Hypertension Society Guidelines for Hypertension Management[5]
> - Joint British Societies' Guidelines-2 (JBS-2) for the Primary Prevention of Cardiovascular Disease in Clinical Practice[6]
> - National Service Framework for Coronary Heart Disease (England) www.nelh.nhs/uk/nsf/chd/nsf
> - Scottish Intercollegiate Guidelines Network (SIGN) www.sign.ac.uk
> - National Assembly for Wales, Tackling CHD in Wales: Implementing Through Evidence; www.wales.nhs.uk/publications/coronary-heart-disease-e.pdf
> - Clinical Resource Efficiency Support Team (CREST) (Northern Ireland) www.crestni.org.uk
>
> **Europe**
> - Recommendations of the European Society of Cardiology (ESC)[7] www.escardio.org
>
> **USA**
> - Recommendations of the Third Report of the National Cholesterol Education Program Adult Treatment Panel (NCEP ATP III)[8] www.nhlbi.nih.gov/guidelines/cholesterol/atp_iii.htm

total and LDL-cholesterol are reached. Other trials completed (PROVE-IT, TNT) or in progress (IDEAL, SEARCH) are specifically designed to explore whether treatment targets should be reduced even further (*see Qs 8.4–8.7*).

In 2004, the NCEP published modifications to the Adult Treatment Panel III guidelines to incorporate the implications of clinical trials published since 2001.[9] An LDL-cholesterol target of <1.8 mmol/L (<70 mg/dL) was proposed as an optional therapeutic target for patients at 'very high risk' or if baseline LDL-cholesterol was <2.6 mmol/L (<100 mg/dL). 'Very high risk' is defined as patients with established cardiovascular disease with:

- multiple major risk factors (especially diabetes)
- severe/poorly controlled risk factors (especially smoking)
- multiple risk factors of the metabolic syndrome
- acute coronary syndromes.

9.6 What are the pros and cons of targets?

Lipid targets are extrapolated from the evidence base of clinical trials and provide surrogate goals from which the outcome benefits shown in the

TABLE 9.1 Target lipid levels of consensus guidelines

Guideline	Total cholesterol target (mmol/L)	LDL-cholesterol target (mmol/L)	Comments
Joint British Societies-2	<4 or 25% reduction	<2 or 30% reduction	Whichever is greater
National Service Framework for Coronary Heart Disease	<5.0	<3.0	Audit standard
Scottish Intercollegiate Guidelines Network	<5.0 or 20–25% reduction	<3.0 or 30% reduction	Whichever is greater
National Assembly for Wales	<5.0 or 2 mmol/L reduction	<3.0	
Clinical Resource Efficiency Support Team (CREST)	<5.0	<3.0	
European Society of Cardiology	<4.5	<2.5	In general In established cardiovascular disease and diabetes
National Cholesterol Education Program (ATP III)		<1.8	Optional in very high risk patients
		<2.6	CHD, CHD equivalents, 10-year CHD risk >20%
		<3.4	2+ risk factors, 10-year CHD risk <20%
		<4.2	0–1 risk factors
			(all LDL-cholesterol reductions to be 30–40%)

CHD, coronary heart disease.

trials should be delivered. Both health professionals and patients feel comfortable with a goal of therapy (especially if this is simple and easy to remember) and target levels can be a powerful aid to fostering compliance.

As a driver to implementation, achieving target lipid levels in a population at high risk is likely to achieve a powerful mass effect and this is why cholesterol targets have been incorporated as quality markers in the new GMS contract for GPs in the UK.

It should be remembered that guideline targets are based on expert consensus agreement and have not been tested a priori by clinical trials. Very few outcome trials have tested the appropriateness of the targets (4S, GREACE and the POST CABG trials are exceptions). In addition, the production of guidelines from different consensus bodies inevitably generates confusion among clinicians with different targets, different target values and varying degrees of complexity to apply.

For many health professionals, measurement difficulties mean LDL-cholesterol is a difficult target to monitor. Percentage reduction targets rather than absolute target values have some merit as they are directly based on the percentage cholesterol reductions observed in the landmark trials but they are difficult to calculate and pose coding difficulties for audit systems.

Lastly, targets (which are designed for the majority) are not always appropriate for the individual and can lead to complacency. Examples based on a total cholesterol target of <5.0 mmol/L (the GMS target) where more aggressive therapy is indicated include:

- the patient who has a myocardial infarction (MI) with a total cholesterol of 4.9 mmol/L
- the patient who has an MI with a total cholesterol of 5.1 mmol/L who achieves a treatment value of 4.9 mmol/L
- the patient who has an MI who achieves a total cholesterol of 4.9 mmol/L whose LDL-cholesterol is 3.3 mmol/L by virtue of low high density lipoprotein (HDL) cholesterol and raised triglycerides.

By setting lower targets, new guidelines will obviate some of these issues but the same principles will apply.

Based on the premise of the Heart Protection Study, some authorities believe that target lipid levels are unnecessary, pointing out that exposing a high-risk population to 1 mmol/L LDL-cholesterol reduction over 5 years, with simvastatin 40 mg, is associated with a significant reduction in clinical events, irrespective of the achieved cholesterol level.

9.7 Is total cholesterol the best target?

The major cholesterol-lowering trials unequivocally show that reducing cholesterol is associated with a clear reduction in CHD events (*Fig. 9.1*). Trials such as 4S, where the absolute reduction of cholesterol is greater,

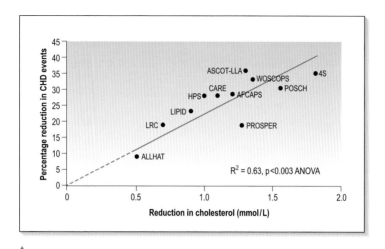

Fig. 9.1 Reduction in coronary heart disease events with lipid-lowering therapy; see Glossary for key to studies. (From Brady & Betteridge,[10] with permission.)

produce proportionately greater benefits than trials such as ALLHAT, where the net absolute reduction in cholesterol was small. Total cholesterol is simple to measure and therefore an appealing target parameter but whether the target should be an absolute concentration (e.g. <5.0 mmol/L) or take into account starting concentrations (with absolute or percentage reductions) remains unsettled.

Although more difficult to measure, LDL-cholesterol is the preferred target. LDL-cholesterol and its physical and chemical modifications are integrally involved in our current understanding of atherosclerosis and when cholesterol is lowered by lipid-lowering therapy, the principal benefit is reduction of LDL-cholesterol. We have already seen an instance where a low level of HDL-cholesterol produces a satisfactory total cholesterol concentration but disguises residual LDL-cholesterol elevation. High levels of HDL-cholesterol can have the opposite effect, with satisfactory LDL-cholesterol levels but apparently inadequate total cholesterol concentrations.

Plotting LDL-cholesterol reduction against CHD risk produces a similar straight-line relationship to that seen for cholesterol in *Figure 9.1*, with every 1% decrease in LDL-cholesterol associated with roughly a 1.25% decrease in

CHD risk. Currently, it seems reasonable to aim for at least a 30% decrease in LDL-cholesterol or an absolute concentration of 2.0 mmol/L, whichever is the lower (*Fig. 9.2*).

For individuals with low HDL-cholesterol or raised triglycerides, achieving total and LDL-cholesterol targets fails to address the total risk conferred by the lipoprotein pattern. European guidelines recognise low HDL-cholesterol (<1.0 mmol/L for men and <1.2 mmol/L for women) and triglycerides <1.7 mmol/L as markers of increased cardiovascular risk but do not set targets. A secondary non-HDL cholesterol goal (of 30 mg/dL lower than the relevant LDL-cholesterol target) is set by NCEP ATP III when triglycerides are raised (>2.3 mmol/L). The new Joint British Societies' guidelines also advocate desirable levels for HDL-cholesterol and triglycerides as well as non-HDL-cholesterol:

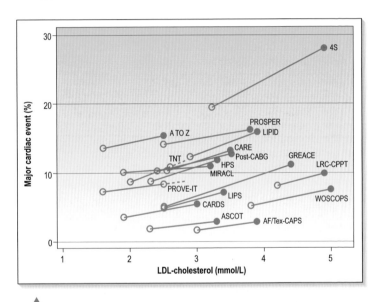

Fig. 9.2 Coronary heart disease rates and LDL-cholesterol levels in placebo and treated patients in major randomised controlled trials of LDL-cholesterol lowering (with statins, except colestyramine in LRC-CPPT). The filled circles repressent the CHD rates and LDL-cholesterol values in the placebo patients, and the open circles the results in the treated groups, lines connecting results in each trial. Whether the studies were higher risk secondary prevention or lower risk primary prevention, and whether the initial LDL-cholesterol levels were higher or lower, benefit was seen. Note that in the more recent trials the achieved LDL-cholesterol values were 2 mmol/L and below. In PROVE-IT and TNT the comparisons are between two active groups of different efficacy without placebo groups.

- triglycerides: <1.7 mmol/L
- HDL-cholesterol: >1.0 mmol/L (men); >1.2 mmol/L (women)
- non-HDL cholesterol: <3.0 mmol/L.

9.8 What is non-HDL-cholesterol?

Non-HDL-cholesterol is calculated by subtracting the concentration of HDL-cholesterol from the concentration of total cholesterol. What is left identifies not only LDL-cholesterol but also triglyceride-rich lipoproteins which are also atherogenic. We have seen the atherogenicity of partially degraded very low density lipoprotein (VLDL), or remnant lipoproteins, in the condition type III dysbetalipoproteinaemia (*see Ch. 4*) and the best measure of their concentration is VLDL-cholesterol. Non-HDL-cholesterol is effectively the sum of LDL-cholesterol and VLDL-cholesterol.

The NCEP ATP III recognises non-HDL-cholesterol as a secondary target of therapy in individuals with high triglycerides. It is particularly useful in patients with established vascular disease and mixed hyperlipidaemia. The NCEP goal of therapy is to reduce non-HDL-cholesterol to <3.4 mmol/L. In effect, the goal is set 0.8 mmol/L higher than the LDL-cholesterol goal on the premise that a VLDL-cholesterol level <0.8 mmol/L is normal.

Non-HDL-cholesterol is recognised by the new Joint British Societies' recommendations with a desirable value of <3.0 mmol/L.

9.9 Are target levels attainable?

In 1999, a meta-analysis of the combined results of 4S, CARE, LIPID, WOSCOPS and AFCAPS/TexCAPS showed that it was possible to reduce cholesterol and LDL-cholesterol by 20 and 28% respectively, for long enough to reduce major CHD events by 31% and total mortality by 20%.[11] In GREACE, total cholesterol was reduced by 36% and LDL-cholesterol by 46% in the 'real world' setting of a CHD secondary prevention clinic, with improved outcomes. Efficacy studies for the newest statin, rosuvastatin, show total cholesterol and LDL-cholesterol reductions up to double those seen in the 1999 meta-analysis. Finally, the addition of ezetimibe to a statin (*see Q 7.31*) offers the possibility of lowering LDL-cholesterol even further and the combination of atorvastatin 80 mg and ezetimibe 10 mg has been shown to lower LDL-cholesterol by around 60%.

With this sort of armamentarium the practitioner can get the majority of patients to target. This contrasts with the situation in the management of both hypertension and diabetes where, despite multiple therapies, target failure is commonplace. Drugs for blood pressure and glycaemic control are less effective and are often associated with adverse effects which limit their use. By and large, lipid-lowering drugs are well tolerated and patient compliance is better.

There will be occasions when it proves impossible to reach lipid targets. Reducing LDL-cholesterol from 6.0 to 3.6 mmol/L represents a 40% reduction in the absolute concentration and a 50% reduction in the CHD risk yet is technically a target failure. It must be remembered that guidelines emphasise ideal practice but a commonsense attitude to non-achievement should prevail and neither practitioner nor patient should be made to feel a failure.

9.10 What are the strategies to achieve target lipid levels?

National recommendations backed by new contractual arrangements for primary care, where the achievement of lipid-lowering standards will be financially rewarded, will focus the minds of primary care professionals on cholesterol targets. Having ensured that the patient is eating healthily and compliant with medication, the four strategies to achieve lipid targets are:

- *Titration*: this traditional approach has been a manifest failure as patients tend to stay on low (often starter) doses of drugs and, for a number of reasons, fail to be titrated upwards.
- '*Right first time*': using a drug that is efficacious enough to get most patients to target at the chosen starter dose. This is more agreeable to the patient, though some will still need titration.
- *Switching*: if an inadequate response is found with one drug, switching to a more effective one.
- *Combination therapy*: adding a second drug with a different mechanism of action to produce a complementary response. Most combinations involve a statin with a fibrate, or a resin, ezetimibe, fish oil or nicotinic acid (*see Ch. 7*).

9.11 How often should lipids be checked once at target?

Tachyphylaxis (a lessening of effect with time) has not been seen with lipid-lowering drugs and, given good compliance with drugs and lifestyle, benefits to the lipid profile should be maintained. Most authorities recommend annual checking for compliance purposes once targets are achieved and this is easy to build into structures of care. The new GP contract in the UK allows total cholesterol measurements recorded over the preceding 15 months.

9.12 How important is global risk factor modification?

Most cardiovascular events occur in individuals with 'average' rather than extreme levels of risk factors, firstly because 'average' levels of risk factors are more common and secondly because, even at 'average' levels, interaction promotes cardiovascular risk. In a population where cholesterol levels are high (such as the UK), CHD events occur more frequently where cholesterol levels are average. One of the reasons for the failure of clinicians to implement lipid-lowering treatment is a failure to appreciate the amount that cholesterol contributes to risk even at ostensibly lower levels. There is now considerable evidence from the statin trials, particularly the HPS, that lowering cholesterol in high-risk individuals, irrespective of the initial concentration, will lessen the likelihood of a cardiovascular event. A parallel finding is seen in the secondary prevention of stroke in the PROGRESS trial where, regardless of baseline blood pressure, treatment with perindopril and indapamide reduced the chance of a further event.[12]

In the lipid-lowering arm of the ASCOT study, the benefits of adding lipid-lowering treatment to subjects with well-controlled blood pressure (138/80 mmHg), whose average cholesterol was only 5.5 mmol/L, included a further 36% reduction in the risk of CHD and a 27% reduction in the risk of stroke.

The concept of global risk reduction has been taken further by Wald and Law who propose that a composite 'polypill' containing aspirin, a statin, three anti-hypertensives in half-dose and folic acid should be taken by all those with vascular disease and those aged over 55 years.[13] By their calculations the synthesis of the benefits would reduce CHD events by 88% and stroke by 80%, although commentators have disputed the particular components of the pill and highlighted issues of multiple real or perceived side effects.

9.13 How common is poor compliance?

Poor compliance is clearly one of the factors responsible for the 'implementation gap' between the evidence base and actual clinical practice. The true extent of non-compliance or non-persistence with prescribed lipid-lowering therapy is unknown but small surveys suggest that after 1 year, barely 50% of patients continue their medication, a finding in line with the experience of other long-term treatments, such as anti-hypertensive drugs.

Technically, a distinction should be made between full non-compliance and partial compliance. Partial compliance is invariably the rule and, overall, patients take only three-quarters of medication prescribed. The most common reasons cited include:

- lack of planning
- forgetfulness
- altered daily schedule
- confused instructions
- lack of efficacy (real or perceived)
- adverse effects.

9.14 What can be done to improve compliance?

Compliance is known to improve both before and after an encounter with a health professional. This emphasises the potential of ongoing support by an interested health professional with their patient. The American National Cholesterol Education Program (NCEP) lists helpful tactics for enhancing compliance (*Box 9.2*). The role of 'expert patients' needs evaluation.

9.15 Who should be referred to a specialist lipid clinic?

The impetus of national initiatives highlighting the importance of lipid modification, the sheer number of people involved and the continuous nature of therapy mean that lipid management is fast becoming an everyday primary care discipline. Most patients with dyslipidaemia can be investigated and treated effectively in primary care without referral to a specialist but, paradoxically, the increasing patient burden means an enhanced role for the specialist lipidologist as well.

BOX 9.2 Tactics to enhance compliance with lipid-lowering treatment

- Teach the patient about the treatment regimen – instructions should be simple but comprehensive
- Help the patient to remember to take the medication – tailor doses to daily habits
- Reinforce compliance – ask about it, chart lipid responses, provide encouragement
- Anticipate common problems and teach the patient how to manage them
- Involve a family member or friend in the patient's therapy programme
- Establish a supportive relationship with the patient – provide ongoing updates and information about the patient's illness and treatment
- Provide individualised services for patients who avoid compliance
- Assess barriers
  — physical (e.g. poor vision, forgetfulness)
  — access (e.g. transportation, income and time)
  — attitude (e.g. fatalism)
  — therapy (e.g. complexity and real or perceived side effects)
  — social (e.g. family instability)
  — faulty perceptions (e.g. denial)

Patients who should be referred to a specialist lipid clinic include the following:

■ *Those who fail to show an effective response to treatment* (whether by virtue of the type and severity of their dyslipidaemia or their intolerance of first line agents)

■ *Those with extreme values* (practitioners often feel less secure with mixed hyperlipidaemia and hypertriglyceridaemia than pure hypercholesterolaemia)

■ *Those with familial dyslipidaemia* (e.g. familial hypercholesterolaemia, familial combined hypercholesterolaemia and types I, III and V, should be managed by specialists as family tracking may be easier to coordinate, drug doses used are higher and combination therapies are more common)

■ *Special cases* (e.g. those requiring the help of joint paediatric, nephrology, neurology, vascular surgery and HIV clinics, hyperlipidaemia associated with poor diabetic control, or those requiring special investigations such as apolipoproteins, enzyme testing, DNA genotyping or more detailed vascular assessment).

9.16 Why have statins been made available 'over the counter'?

It is clear that more people need to be on statins. Although they have been available for 15 years and have a proven track record of benefit and safety, the majority of patients who have either experienced an atherosclerotic event or who are at high risk of one are still not receiving treatment. The reasons for this are discussed in *Question 9.2*. For those at moderate risk, who would not qualify for routine prescription, low-dose statin status has been reclassified, allowing their supervision by a pharmacist. There is evidence that lipid management services provided by community pharmacists can enhance the prescribing and use of lipid-lowering drugs, help patients reach target levels and reduce cardiovascular risk. Amidst world-wide scrutiny, the UK government sanctioned the availability of simvastatin 10 mg 'over the counter' (OTC) from July 2004.

In the UK, nearly five million people under 70 would qualify for statin treatment using the latest thresholds for intervention. Government predictions in the UK project statin costs to £2.1 billion by 2010, even taking into account patent expiries for the majority of the class. The evidence base, however, shows that statins are effective even in populations at low overall cardiovascular risk (e.g. AFCAPS/TexCAPS), albeit with lower absolute benefit. Making statins available OTC means that individuals at moderate risk, who are just below the intervention threshold (i.e. 10–20% 10-year cardiovascular event risk), can benefit from cardiovascular risk reduction if they so choose and at their own expense.

9.17 What are the concerns surrounding 'over-the-counter' statins?

Any drug considered for OTC use must have a good safety profile. The incidence of adverse effects with statins both from clinical trials and experiential reporting is very low. Physicians, however, are nervous of the potential of liver and muscle damage and transmit these concerns to patients (*see Q 7.6*).

Other concerns regarding OTC statin use are outlined in *Box 9.3*.

BOX 9.3 Additional issues regarding over-the-counter statin use

- Heightened social inequality with use by the more affluent
- Inappropriate use if protocol not followed
- Using the statin as an alternative to lifestyle changes
- 'Upstream' pressures on primary care services to monitor treatment, deal with side effects or prescribe at lower than recommended thresholds
- Inadequate risk assessment and management of other risk factors by pharmacists
- Inadequate treatment of more severe lipid disorders (e.g. missing the diagnosis of familial hypercholesterolaemia and the opportunity of family tracing)
- Continuing compliance – a consumer support programme is essential
- Poor communication with general practitioners who may not be aware their patient is taking a statin
- The need for sufficient evaluation and quality assurance of the process and outcomes

---

PATIENT QUESTION

9.18 Who should take 'over-the-counter' statins?

Individuals who are likely to benefit from OTC statins are those with a 10-year cardiovascular event risk of approximately 10–20% (the orange band of the Joint British Societies risk prediction charts; *see Fig. 5.1*). Roughly speaking, this level of risk applies to:

- men >55 years
- men aged 45–55 years or women >55 years who:
    — have a family history of coronary heart disease, or
    — smoke, or
    — are overweight, or
    — are of South Asian origin.

The pharmacist will advise you to be managed by your doctor if you have already been diagnosed with coronary heart disease, stroke, peripheral arterial disease, very high inherited cholesterol, diabetes, high blood pressure or impaired kidney function. In addition, the pharmacist will check for potential drug interactions and that certain contraindications (such as statin allergy, liver disease or excess alcohol consumption, porphyria, pregnancy or breastfeeding) are not apparent.

Although blood cholesterol tests are not mandatory, these are available via the pharmacy and are recommended to enhance risk assessment and monitor the effects of treatment. A comprehensive support and education package is available to advise consumers on all aspects of cardiovascular disease prevention (see www.jnjmsd.co.uk/zocor/).

Special situations

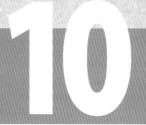

10.1	Is it safe to give lipid-lowering drugs to children with hyperlipidaemia?	156
10.2	How effective are statins in older people?	156
10.3	Is lipid-lowering treatment as effective in women as in men?	157
10.4	Can women with familial hypercholesterolaemia take the oral contraceptive pill?	157
10.5	Can lipid-lowering drugs be taken in pregnancy?	158
10.6	What are the effects of hormone replacement therapy on lipids?	159
10.7	What is the role of lipid lowering for the patient with hypertension?	159
10.8	What is the role of lipid lowering for the patient with diabetes?	161
10.9	What is the role of lipid lowering for the patient with peripheral arterial disease?	162
10.10	What is the role of lipid lowering for the patient with chronic renal disease?	162
10.11	What is the role of lipid lowering for the patient with HIV?	163
10.12	What is the role of lipid lowering for the patient with a stroke?	163
10.13	What is the role of lipid lowering for the patient with heart failure?	164

PQ PATIENT QUESTIONS

10.14	Can you be too old for lipid-lowering treatment?	165
10.15	Do statins prevent dementia?	165
10.16	Does treatment for blood pressure affect lipid levels?	165
10.17	Do statins prevent osteoporosis?	166

10.1 Is it safe to give lipid-lowering drugs to children with hyperlipidaemia?

Some genetic hyperlipidaemias, such as familial hypercholesterolaemia (FH), are expressed from birth and affected children have impaired endothelial function and the early lesions of atherosclerosis from an early age. In contrast, familial combined hyperlipidaemia tends to be identifiable in young adults in affected families.

The mainstay of treatment is a low fat diet, which is safe as long as overall calorie intake is sufficient and this can be commenced from 2 years of age.

The use of medication is a matter of judgement. In a child where there is a family history of coronary heart disease (CHD) in the third decade, it might be reasonable to start medication at 10 years of age. Girls with FH are less likely to require medication as early unless there is a pattern of early CHD in a female relative. The anion exchange resins have been the drugs of choice but compliance is poor. Although without long-term safety data in children, statins are increasingly used and in America Stein et al showed that lovastatin reduced low density lipoprotein (LDL) cholesterol in adolescent boys with FH by 27%, without compromising growth, hormonal or other nutritional factors.[1] A recent Dutch study in 214 children, aged 8–18 years, with familial hypercholesterolaemia showed significant carotid intima-media thickness differences in those treated with pravastatin without any observed differences in growth, muscle or liver enzyme levels or parameters of endocrine function.[2]

Children with inherited hyperlipidaemia also need general advice on a healthy lifestyle with the accent on increased physical activity and not smoking.

10.2 How effective are statins in older people?

Epidemiological studies show that the association between cholesterol and CHD decreases with age. Despite this, because the burden of CHD increases with age, the risk attributable to cholesterol actually increases and measures to reduce cholesterol in older people are potentially highly effective.

The issue was not clarified by the earlier statin trials which were largely conducted in middle-aged men, but subgroup analysis nevertheless suggested equivalent benefit for older subjects. The Heart Protection Study (HPS) and PROSPER[3] recruited patients between 40 and 80 and 70 and 82 years respectively, meaning that, with follow-up, we now have data to

85 years. In the 1263 patients aged between 75 and 80 years at recruitment in HPS, major vascular events were highly significantly reduced by nearly a third. In PROSPER, LDL-cholesterol was reduced by 34% and the end point of fatal and non-fatal myocardial infarction/cerebrovascular accident by 15%. Despite this apparent LDL-cholesterol effect, those individuals in the lowest tertile for high density lipoprotein (HDL) cholesterol gained the most benefit and those with an LDL-cholesterol to HDL-cholesterol ratio >3 accounted for most of the pravastatin action. Translating these relative benefits into a population at high absolute risk of vascular disease is likely to be highly cost effective.

There are very close parallels to the evolution of the use of statins in older people and the gradual definition of the role of antihypertensive therapy in the elderly over the last 25 years.

10.3 Is lipid-lowering treatment as effective in women as in men?

For many years, the erroneous perception that vascular disease was chiefly a problem for men and the low event rates in younger women meant that few women were recruited for clinical trials involving lipid-lowering therapy. It is now clear that, while the onset of vascular disease in women is commonly delayed by about 10 years compared to men, after 65 years the rates are more equal and the same risk factors are operative. Indeed, women tend to have higher levels of total and LDL-cholesterol, triglycerides and fibrinogen and an increased prevalence of obesity, diabetes and hypertension. Offsetting this are lower levels of smoking, reduced central obesity and higher levels of HDL-cholesterol. Women with diabetes lose their relative cardiovascular disease (CVD) protection.

Although under-represented in the main outcome trials of cholesterol lowering, the benefits in women generally equalled, or even exceeded, those seen in men (*Table 10.1*). The Heart Protection Study deliberately recruited larger numbers of older and female patients and conclusively demonstrated equivalent major vascular event reduction (367:450 [active:placebo] in 5082 female subjects) in women as well as in men, and removed any lingering doubts about the efficacy of lipid-lowering therapy in women at cardiovascular risk.

10.4 Can women with familial hypercholesterolaemia take the oral contraceptive pill?

There has been much debate about the possible harmful effects of the oral contraceptive pill and this is particularly relevant to higher risk women. Early reports identified hazards with higher doses of oestrogen but as these

TABLE 10.1 CHD events in primary and secondary statin trials in women

| Trial | Treatment | | Control | | |
	CHD events	No. of patients	CHD events	No. of patients	Odds ratio
AFCAPS/TexCAPS	7	499	13	498	0.54 (ns)
4S	59	407	91	420	0.62
CARE	46	286	80	290	0.51
LIPID	90	756	104	760	0.85 (ns)

CHD, coronary heart disease; ns, not significant.

were reduced, the progestin component came under scrutiny. While oestrogens raise very low density lipoprotein (VLDL) cholesterol and HDL-cholesterol they can also lower LDL-cholesterol. In contrast, progestins lower HDL-cholesterol and raise LDL-cholesterol. In addition, because of their glucocorticoid and mineralocorticoid effects, both oestrogens and progestins tend to impair glucose tolerance and raise blood pressure.

As with all women, each case should be assessed individually. In the absence of hypertension, diabetes and obesity it is safe for women with familial hypercholesterolaemia to take a modern low dose formulation, at least to 35 years of age. The most important thing is not to smoke.

10.5 Can lipid-lowering drugs be taken in pregnancy?

In practice, the question whether to continue lipid-lowering therapy in pregnancy arises in relatively few women, usually with identified genetic or diabetic dyslipidaemia. In pregnancy, total cholesterol and LDL-cholesterol levels rise towards term by about 30% and remain elevated for at least 8 weeks postnatally. The biggest rise is seen in triglycerides which increase two- to three-fold (albeit that pancreatitis is rare and usually associated with biliary disease, an underlying mixed hyperlipidaemia and/or diabetes). HDL-cholesterol increases in early pregnancy but falls in the third trimester.

 The safety of statins and fibrates is not established in pregnancy and the recommendations are that these drugs should be stopped prior to conception if possible and certainly when pregnancy is identified. They can be resumed at the end of breast feeding and treatment does not have to be limited in men wishing to father children. The non-absorbed bile acid sequestrant resins and fish oils are not contraindicated in pregnancy.

One report of 134 women inadvertently exposed to lovastatin or simvastatin showed no adverse foetal outcome[4] but a recent study from the US National Institutes of Health[5] found that of 52 babies exposed to statins in the first trimester of pregnancy, 20 were born with central nervous system defects and limb deformities.

10.6 What are the effects of hormone replacement therapy on lipids?

The menopause sees an increase in total and LDL-cholesterol, triglycerides and lipoprotein(a) (Lp(a)). HDL-cholesterol is slightly reduced but this disguises a proportionately greater reduction in the more protective HDL_2 subclass. Adding oestrogen reverses these changes but when progestins must be used for endometrial protection some of the oestrogen benefits are opposed. Nevertheless, the approximate net effects of combined HRT are to reduce total cholesterol by 8%, LDL-cholesterol by 14% and Lp(a) by 19%, while increasing HDL-cholesterol by 11% and triglycerides by 13%. The rise in triglycerides is seen with oral preparations only and is reversed by using transdermal administration.

In the 1990s, the changes in the lipoprotein profile induced by hormone replacement therapy (HRT) seemed to offer the most plausible explanation for the 30–40% reduction in CHD events seen in HRT users in early USA observational studies. To remove the effects of bias, intervention trials were needed to confirm the benefits of HRT and it came as a major shock to clinicians when secondary prevention trials such as HERS and ERA failed to deliver outcome benefits despite achieving the predicted changes in lipid levels. The definitive Women's Health Initiative trial was stopped 3 years early in 2002 when it became apparent that the risks of treatment exceeded the benefits.[6] In 16 608 women (mean age 63.3 years) taking combined HRT the risk of myocardial infarction (MI) and death was 24% higher than in women taking placebo. As far as the individual is concerned, the risk is still low (39 cases of CHD per 100 000 women against 33 per 100 000) but coupled with increased rates of stroke, venous thromboembolism and breast cancer (verified by the Million Women Study) the findings have led to a complete reappraisal of the use of HRT. *Authorities now agree limited exposure related to menopausal symptom severity and not cardiovascular disease or osteoporosis prevention.*

In the future, selective oestrogen receptor modulators (SERMs) may offer hope and both raloxifene and tamoxifen have been examined for their effects on cardiovascular risk factors. Again, both produce favourable effects on the lipid profile but women using tamoxifen in the Breast Cancer Prevention Trial showed no reduction in CHD.

10.7 What is the role of lipid lowering for the patient with hypertension?

Trials of antihypertensive therapy have demonstrated unequivocal benefit in terms of stroke reduction but the impact on CHD (which is a much more significant cause of death and morbidity) has been less impressive. Several explanations have been put forward to explain this discrepancy. A simple answer may be that the blood pressure lowering achieved in the trials has been inadequate in terms of degree or duration. In addition, as CHD is a multifactorial disease and as risk factors cluster together in high-risk individuals, attention to a single risk factor does little in terms of reducing overall global risk. Finally, it has been proposed that adverse metabolic effects of the antihypertensive drugs themselves may curtail their outcome benefits.

Antihypertensives with adverse metabolic effects produce more marked changes where dyslipidaemia or impaired glucose tolerance already exist. Thiazides and beta-blockers (particularly of the non-selective kind) tend to increase total and LDL-cholesterol, reduce HDL-cholesterol and elevate triglycerides. New guidelines from the British Hypertension Society reflect growing appreciation of the diabetogenic potential of these drugs, particularly in combination, and promote the roles of newer agents.[7,8] Angiotensin converting enzyme (ACE) inhibitors, angiotensin receptor blockers and calcium antagonists are lipid neutral whereas alpha blockers often improve the lipid profile with small reductions in LDL-cholesterol and triglycerides and a small rise in HDL-cholesterol.

Subgroup analyses of all the major statin trials show that hypertensive patients derive similar benefits to non-hypertensives. As befits the global risk modification of modern hypertension management, two major new hypertension trials – ALLHAT[9] and ASCOT[10] – have included lipid-lowering arms. ALLHAT proved disappointing with a non-significant 9% reduction in the 6-year CHD event rate due to a modest intergroup difference in LDL-cholesterol as a result of non-adherence to the study statin (pravastatin) and crossover to other therapies. In contrast, the lipid-lowering arm of ASCOT was stopped early when interim analysis showed a 36% reduction in CHD and a 27% reduction in stroke in optimally treated hypertensives (mean BP 138/80 mmHg) with cholesterol <6.5 mmol/L who took atorvastatin 10 mg.

All new guidelines emphasise the need for global risk modification in individuals whose 10-year CHD risk exceeds 15%. This is equivalent to a 20% 10-year cardiovascular risk or a 5% 10-year risk of cardiovascular death. Inevitably, this will mean the majority of hypertensives will need composite treatment with lipid-lowering agents as well as antihypertensive and antiplatelet therapy.

10.8 What is the role of lipid lowering for the patient with diabetes?

Cardiovascular disease is the most common complication of diabetes. While there is some heterogeneity, people with diabetes approach the same CHD risk as people without diabetes who have had a heart attack. Stroke is increased two-fold, transient ischaemic attack (TIA) two- to six-fold and the chance of lower limb amputation is 15- to 40-fold that of the general population. In type 2 diabetes, the evidence for modifying risk factors such as cholesterol and blood pressure is strong, whereas intensive management of glycaemia only reduces microvascular (not macrovascular) outcomes significantly.[11] As a result, the presence of diabetes is now recognised by all major guidelines to confer an equivalent risk to that of secondary prevention, and treatment with lipid-lowering drugs is recommended.

Dyslipidaemia is common in diabetic populations and is characterised by moderate hypertriglyceridaemia and low HDL-cholesterol concentrations. Total and LDL-cholesterol concentrations are similar to non-diabetic populations but LDL-cholesterol tends qualitatively towards the small, dense variety.

Sufficient patient numbers were included in the major trials to confirm the benefits of statins in diabetes, establishing LDL-cholesterol reduction as the major therapeutic target, with non-HDL-cholesterol a secondary target. In the HPS, 5963 patients with diabetes were recruited, 3982 of whom had no prior CHD. Major vascular events were reduced (601 vs. 748) by simvastatin, independent of baseline cholesterol. The placebo-controlled Collaborative Atorvastatin Diabetes Study (CARDS) was designed to assess the efficacy of atorvastatin 10 mg daily in the primary prevention of cardiovascular events in 2838 patients with type 2 diabetes, and was stopped 2 years early after 3.9 years, when the risk reductions in the atorvastatin group showed strongly significant benefits. The risk of major cardiovascular events was reduced by 37% and the risk of acute coronary events, coronary revascularisation and stroke by 36, 31 and 48%, respectively.[12]

In diabetic dyslipidaemia, the rationale for fibrate therapy is plausible but evidence of benefit is less consistent. VA-HIT showed a reduction in events with gemfibrozil in the diabetic subgroup but bezafibrate in BIP showed no overall benefit. DAIS, an angiographic trial of fenofibrate in type 2 diabetes, showed significant reduction in atherosclerotic progression and a reduction in clinical events.[13] FIELD is a major clinical outcome study of fenofibrate in 8000 patients with type 2 diabetes and will answer many questions in primary and secondary prevention.

Patients with type 1 diabetes are also at increased risk of vascular disease (especially those with proteinuria and hypertension) but there is less trial evidence to guide the clinician. A powerful case can be made for all patients with diabetes receiving aggressive lipid lowering in conjunction with blood pressure optimisation, antiplatelet therapy and glycaemic control.

10.9 What is the role of lipid lowering for the patient with peripheral arterial disease?

Guidelines for the management of cardiovascular risk and dyslipidaemia include patients with peripheral arterial disease (PAD) in those recommended for priority treatment. This correctly reflects the cross-risk of vascular disease, patients with PAD having a much increased risk of CHD and stroke. The promise of lipid-lowering therapies was shown in an early angiographic study which demonstrated reduced femoral plaque progression but again it was the HPS that confirmed the hypothesis. Simvastatin 40 mg reduced major vascular events (MVEs) in 2701 patients with PAD but no prior CHD (327 vs. 420 MVEs). Given full compliance, the authors estimate that treating 1000 patients at this level of risk for 5 years with simvastatin 40 mg would save 70 MVEs.

More recently, a small study of 354 patients with intermittent claudication highlighted improved lifestyle when treated with atorvastatin, the trial subjects enjoying an increased duration of pain-free walking, a complementary benefit to the expected reduction in cardiovascular events.

The benefits in PAD appear to extend beyond the use of statins. In the LEADER trial of 1568 men with 'lower extremity arterial disease' (mean age 68.2 years), bezafibrate 400 mg was associated with a 62% reduction of CHD in men under (albeit not over) 65 years.[14]

10.10 What is the role of lipid lowering for the patient with chronic renal disease?

It has been known for some time that cardiovascular mortality is increased in haemodialysis patients, with up to a 100-fold excess in younger patients. The pattern is atypical, with fewer patients dying of MI and stroke and relatively more from cardiac arrest, cardiomyopathy and heart failure. Although the observational data are inadequate, they seem to show that raised cholesterol is not associated with the increased risk of death. In addition, the histological pattern of arterial disease is more suggestive of arteriosclerosis, rather than atherosclerosis, with stiffer, more hypertrophied and calcified arteries accounting for increased levels of systolic hypertension and heart failure.

Despite this, the pattern of lipid abnormality commonly seen in patients with chronic renal disease mimics the atherogenic pattern seen in metabolic syndrome (*see* Q 4.3) and type 2 diabetes with modest elevations of total and LDL-cholesterol (much higher in nephrotic syndrome), low HDL-cholesterol and raised triglycerides. In addition, qualitative changes in LDL-cholesterol mean increased levels of small, dense LDL-cholesterol.

Patients with chronic kidney disease have tended to be excluded from clinical trials but there is some information from HPS and ALERT. In the subgroup of 1329 subjects in HPS with elevated creatinine (but <200 mmol/L) the benefit of simvastatin 40 mg was statistically significant (182 vs. 268 MVEs). Significant reductions in cardiac death and non-fatal MI were seen in ALERT, where renal transplant patients on ciclosporin were treated with fluvastatin, 40–80 mg, for 5 years. More information will emerge from the 4D study (using atorvastatin) and SHARP (using combination treatment with simvastatin and ezetimibe).

Given the current level of evidence, statins are increasingly used in patients with chronic renal disease. Fibrates are generally contraindicated. Care must be taken, especially with ciclosporin, where lower doses of nearly all statins should be used to avoid higher plasma levels and the risk of rhabdomyolysis.

10.11 What is the role of lipid lowering for the patient with HIV?

Highly active antiretroviral therapy (HAART) can be extremely effective in reducing viral load but some of the drugs used are associated with dyslipidaemia. With protease inhibitors, total cholesterol may rise 30–40%, HDL-cholesterol may fall and triglycerides may increase by 200%, sometimes to dangerous levels. The changes are more severe in those individuals who develop lipodystrophy, where lipoatrophy affects the face, limbs and upper chest, with fat accumulation at the back of the neck and around the abdomen. Given the successes of retroviral therapy, patients have now swapped the risks of their infection for the chronic risks of dyslipidaemia and glucose intolerance.

Very high triglyceride levels may be treated with a low fat/low carbohydrate diet, weight reduction, alcohol avoidance, omega-3 fatty acids and fibrates. The more typical dyslipidaemia responds well to statins but as protease inhibitors inhibit cytochrome 3A4, it is probably better to avoid statins metabolised through this route.

10.12 What is the role of lipid lowering for the patient with a stroke?

For many years, observational studies discounted the relationship between cholesterol and stroke, but once haemorrhagic strokes are taken out of the equation, a clear relationship emerges.

For many, it was a surprise when the secondary prevention statin trials began to report reductions in stroke in patients being treated for CHD. 4S showed a reduction in stroke of 29%, CARE, 31% and LIPID, 19%. HPS confirmed the benefit of statins in high-risk patients with 444 strokes in

simvastatin-treated patients compared to 585 in those placebo allocated
(−25%). In addition, TIAs were reduced and there was no excess of
haemorrhagic stroke which had been a concern of cholesterol lowering in
the past. In HPS, 1820 patients with a history of cerebrovascular disease (but
no prior CHD) were randomised and again they showed significant benefits
in MVE reduction (172 vs. 212).

> If atherosclerosis is considered to be a pan-vascular disease,
> reduction in cross-risk between its various manifestations by therapy
> which slows progression and stabilises plaques is easy to understand.

Although the evidence base for statins in the management of
atherothrombotic stroke is accumulating, more information is expected
from SPARCL, a study using atorvastatin in patients with a minor stroke or
TIA, with the primary outcome measure being the effect on total stroke.

10.13 What is the role of lipid lowering for the patient with heart failure?

Some of the major trials of cholesterol lowering have recorded outcome
benefits in heart failure parameters (*Table 10.2*).

Unfortunately, no definitive trial has looked at the question of whether
patients with heart failure benefit from cholesterol lowering. The CARE trial
specifically identified patients with reduced ventricular function (LVEF
<40%) and a reduction in major coronary events was seen (84 vs. 112).
Indirect data from heart failure surveys and trials (e.g. ELITE 2) show that
the death rate in patients treated with a statin is less than those treated
without. In severe heart failure – New York Heart Association (NYHA)
stage 3 or 4 – likely patient longevity may be too short to warrant statin
treatment.

The hypothesis that cholesterol lowering might be helpful in heart
failure derives from the observations that CHD is the cause of heart failure
in about two-thirds of subjects and about one-third of patients with heart

TABLE 10.2 Heart failure development, deaths and hospitalisation in lipid-lowering trials

	Trial	Event type	Events on treatment	Events on placebo	Significance (p)
Statins	4S	New cases	184	228	<0.015
		Deaths	47	73	0.014
	GREACE	Hospitalisation	11	23	0.006
Fibrates	VA-HIT	Hospitalisation	134	168	0.04

failure die of another heart attack. Preventing further CHD events for an individual with heart failure is therefore a key strategy to reduce death.

Concern has been expressed that lowering blood cholesterol in heart failure could be detrimental. Low cholesterol concentrations actually predict a worse outcome in heart failure but this probably reflects low hepatic synthesis in the most severely affected cases.

 PATIENT QUESTIONS

10.14   Can you be too old for lipid-lowering treatment?

As outlined in *Question 10.2*, clinical trials suggest benefit from statins at least up to the age of 80 and probably 85 years. These trials, however, were conducted in individuals at high risk and often with declared disease, such as heart attacks or strokes. For these people, with a reasonable chance of 3 years' longevity, it is probably not too late to start treatment but in terms of primary prevention (*see Ch. 5*) the predictive value of cholesterol concentrations diminishes with age and the position is less clear. There is limited information from primary prevention trials on those aged over 75 years (*see Q 10.2*).

Important additional issues for older people to address with their doctors when considering starting lipid-lowering therapy include lowering the threshold for intervention for favourable biological age, the presence and influence of concomitant illness, life expectancy and the potential dangers of polypharmacy and drug interactions.

10.15   Do statins prevent dementia?

Increasing evidence suggests that atherosclerosis is a major contributor to cognitive decline, largely as a result of the accumulation of multiple episodes of vascular damage to the brain substance. Observational studies that linked statin therapy with a reduced risk of dementia of up to 70% were widely publicised. However, observational studies can easily be biased and the findings need to be confirmed by clinical trials. Two trials, PROSPER and HPS, have examined the question over 3 and 5 years respectively and both showed clearly that cognitive function declined at the same rate in individuals taking statins as those who did not.

10.16   Does treatment for blood pressure affect lipid levels?

Clinical trials of blood pressure lowering drugs have demonstrated unequivocal benefit in terms of stroke reduction but the impact on preventing heart attacks has been less impressive. One of the reasons put forward is the fact that some of the drugs used in the trials have unfavourable effects on the lipid profile.

An analysis of 474 trials where blood pressure drugs were used and lipid levels were checked showed that:

- thiazide diuretics can increase cholesterol and triglycerides by up to 0.3 mmol/L and also slightly reduce HDL-cholesterol
- beta-blockers can increase triglycerides by up to 0.7 mmol/L and reduce HDL-cholesterol by up to 0.1 mmol/L.

Nowadays doctors tend to use lower doses of thiazides and more modern beta-blockers and the adverse effects are probably minimised. Nevertheless, in the ASCOT study[8] there were CVD outcome benefits for ACE-inhibition and calcium channel blockade (perindopril and amlodipine) compared to thiazide diuretics and beta-blockade, while excess new diabetes was seen with the latter treatments in both ASCOT and ALL-HAT[9] studies. Doctors often prescribe other blood pressure drugs first-line where problems with the lipid profile or glucose metabolism already exist. ACE inhibitors, angiotensin receptor blockers and calcium antagonists are lipid neutral and alpha-blockers even have small beneficial effects.

10.17 Do statins prevent osteoporosis?

In 1999 it was shown that administering simvastatin to castrated female rats stimulated the development of bone. Within a year, several studies had shown a reduction of osteoporotic fractures in women over 60 who were taking statins. One study from Korea showed an increase in hip bone density in 36 women who had used statins over the previous 15 months. If validated, the findings would have enormous implications for women's health.

Once again randomised clinical trials are needed. Retrospective analysis of LIPID and HPS and informal communications from the 4S investigators show no reduction in the rate of fractures during the limited duration of the trials and offer no support for the hypothesis.

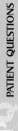

Economic aspects

11

11.1	What are the numbers needed to treat from the major lipid trials?	168
11.2	What is the cost-effectiveness of secondary prevention in coronary heart disease?	169
11.3	What is the cost-effectiveness of primary prevention at different intervention thresholds?	169

PQ PATIENT QUESTION

11.4	How can we afford lipid-lowering therapy?	170

11.1 What are the numbers needed to treat from the major lipid trials?

The concept of the 'number needed to treat' (NNT) is often used by health professionals to gauge the impact of an intervention. The numbers are calculated from the evidence of outcome event trials using the formula:

$$1/\text{absolute risk reduction}$$

or

$$1/\text{control event rate} - \text{treatment event rate.}$$

NNTs should be used with caution as the figures can be presented differently according to which events are being reported and over what period. The focus is usually on non-fatal and fatal coronary heart disease (CHD) and the reduction in other events such as stroke is often not included. In the lipid trials, NNTs for fatal events alone tend to be high and mask considerable morbidity benefits in terms of reducing non-fatal events, revascularisations, hospital admissions and the progression towards more serious disease. In addition, NNTs are not expressed with conventional statistical limits of uncertainty, such as confidence intervals. NNTs for the major statin trials are shown in *Table 11.1*.

NNTs reduce if the baseline absolute risk of the group under investigation increases. For example, in CARE, the 5-year NNT for the diabetic subgroup reduces to 12 and in the 65–75 age range, to 11. Similarly, if the 40% of higher risk WOSCOPS men, whose absolute 10-year CHD risk is ≥20%, are identified, the NNT becomes 22.

TABLE 11.1 Numbers needed to treat derived from the major statin trials

Trial	Events prevented	Placebo (%)*	NNT	Follow-up (years)
WOSCOPS	NF MI/CHD death	8.0	45	4.9
AFCAPS/TexCAPS	NF/F MI UA CHD death	5.5	50	5.2
4S	NF MI/CHD death	25.0	12	5.4
CARE	NF MI/CHD death	13.5	33	5.0
LIPID	NF MI/CHD death	13.0	28	6.1

*Risk rates for placebo groups for events cited in each study, to 5 years. CHD, coronary heart disease; MI, myocardial infarction; NF, non-fatal; NF/F, non-fatal/fatal; NNT, number needed to treat; UA, unstable angina.

11.2 What is the cost-effectiveness of secondary prevention in coronary heart disease?

The 4S study revolutionised the attitudes of clinicians towards statins and well-designed economic evaluations support the clinical evidence. Johannesson et al used the hazard functions from the 4S database to estimate the cost per life year gained for CHD secondary prevention for men and women from 35 to 70 years old.[1] The range was £2375 for a hypercholesterolaemic 70-year-old man to £17 125 for a 35-year-old woman with low cholesterol. When indirect costs (such as lost productivity) were added, treating younger patients was shown to save money.

A second analysis by Jönsson et al incorporated additional data from 4S on reduced hospitalisation costs and calculated that each life year gained cost £5502.[2] Several other studies have confirmed this figure for secondary prevention with minor variations. This is well within the limits of cost-effectiveness normally considered acceptable by sophisticated healthcare systems where interventions are considered highly cost-effective if each life year saved costs <US$20 000. The advent of patent expiries is likely to reduce acquisition costs by at least 50% with corresponding incremental benefits to cost-effectiveness. Indeed, if lifetime (rather than 5–10 year) analyses of cost-effectiveness are carried out, then treatment at CVD rates lower than 10%/10 years may be appropriate.

11.3 What is the cost-effectiveness of primary prevention at different intervention thresholds?

Estimates for cost-effectiveness in primary prevention have proved much more variable. The WOSCOPS investigators calculated the discounted costs per life year gained to be £20 375 across the study population and £13 995 in the higher risk 40%.[3] Other investigators, perhaps with political axes to grind, have inflated the figures significantly. The variations can be accounted for by the use of different methodologies and the failure to incorporate the effects of reductions in other long-term morbidity consequences such as heart failure, stroke and unstable angina. The cost savings involved in stroke reduction alone are significant and are rarely accounted in analyses.

In most studies of the cost-effectiveness of lipid lowering the estimates are based on treatment targeted at threshold concentrations of cholesterol. As cholesterol levels by themselves are poor predictors of risk it is more appropriate to target levels of absolute CHD risk and gross discounted costs per life year gained, including drug costs. Potential savings in healthcare costs for four levels of absolute risk are shown in *Table 11.2*.[4]

In the UK, approximately 4.8% of the adult population requires secondary prevention. Subjects for primary prevention at the 15% CHD (20% CVD) risk level comprise a further 24.7%.[4] *This means that almost 30% of the UK population might require treatment at a cost considerably in excess of £2 billion.* It is difficult to envisage how more aggressive intervention at lower levels of risk will be affordable at current prices in a country with such high levels of CHD risk. Cost-effectiveness is of course country specific and different levels of intervention reflect the political and social pressures of each community on each nation's healthcare system. In the USA, current National Cholesterol Education Program guidelines suggest cholesterol lowering would be applicable for 28% of the population.

TABLE 11.2 Implications of targeting statin treatment at four CHD risk levels, showing the NNT, cost-effectiveness and implications for the UK population

	10-year CHD risk			
	45%	30%	20%	15%
NNT for 5 years	13	20	30	40
Cost per life year gained (£)	5100	8200	10 700	12 500
Percentage of UK adults above threshold	5.1	8.2	15.8	24.7
Annual cost (£millions)	549	885	1712	2673

CHD, coronary heart disease; NNT, number needed to treat.

PATIENT QUESTION

11.4 How can we afford lipid-lowering therapy?

Few medical treatments have received the intensity of cost speculation accorded to lipid-lowering therapy and this is appropriate given the scale of the problem and the potential for benefit. From the outset, to preserve resources, prescribers have been urged to target a certain level of risk, ensure continuous treatment and avoid wasteful prescribing in other therapeutic areas. Most of the drugs prescribed by doctors are for the control of symptoms and relatively few have been shown to both significantly extend life as well as improve its quality.

When the Heart Protection Study was published, the authors said that statins would benefit three times the number of people currently receiving them, not only saving 10 000 lives in the UK, but also reducing non-fatal events, hospital admissions and numerous other healthcare costs. In his report to the UK government in 2002, Wanless predicted a statin spend of £2.1 billion by 2010, assuming treatment at the 15% 10-year CHD risk threshold and 80% compliance. Despite the enormity of this sum, the net cost will be much less than forecast once the benefits are discounted.

On such a massive scale, lipid-lowering therapy is likely to be scarcely achievable in the developed world. In developing countries, whose rate of cardiovascular disease is rising sharply and whose per capita health spend is low, it will be impossible and there is real concern that the issue will magnify health inequalities and divert resources from more relevant health problems.

Some of the concerns about the affordability of lipid lowering are based on short-term views. By 2010, most of the currently available statins will be off patent and in such a large and competitive market their acquisition costs are likely to fall by over 75%. In addition, as statins become available 'over the counter' a significant proportion of the population may self-treat and self-pay.

New horizons – the next 10 years

12

12.1 What are the most exciting basic science issues likely to impact on clinical practice over the next decade?   174

12.2 What new lipid lowering drugs are in the pipeline?   174

12.3 Is gene therapy a realistic possibility?   177

12.4 What are the important scientific issues to be settled by ongoing clinical trials?   178

12.5 What features of clinical guidelines are most likely to change?   179

12.1 What are the most exciting basic science issues likely to impact on clinical practice over the next decade?

In the last few years it has become increasingly clear that the pathology of atherogenesis and atherosclerosis is not a matter of passive lipid deposition in the arterial wall – it is now recognised to be a dynamic picture of recurrent minor damage followed by healing, with chronic inflammation. Much of the time healing leaves only modest residual scarring. The understanding of this process has increased substantially, and the role of multiple vasoactive substances, chemoattractant molecules and cytokines is increasingly understood.

In the next decade we should see this knowledge lead to breakthroughs in our approach to preventing atherogenesis by targeting these core mechanisms. Clearly, the basic repair process that follows arterial damage needs to take place, but excess inflammatory reaction needs to be contained.

In another area, we are seeing increasing understanding of the genetics of atherosclerosis, of the inherited disorders of lipid metabolism, and of inflammation. Gene transfer may become available for disorders such as familial hypercholesterolaemia and for lipoprotein lipase deficiency.

In metabolic syndrome, and obesity, with their cardiovascular consequences, agents such as the thiazolidinediones (which regulate nuclear receptors called PPARs) have shown benefits in improving insulin sensitivity. We need SPPARMs – selective PPAR modulators – without their effects on adipogenesis. More recently cannabinoid receptor blockers working within the brain have shown promise in aiding smoking cessation and in weight reduction to a greater extent than existing agents. To see smoking cessation with weight loss rather than weight gain, and to couple this with improving glucose, insulin, triglyceride and high density lipoprotein (HDL)-cholesterol levels is clearly a major potential therapeutic step. Partial inhibition of the cholesterol ester (and triglyceride) transfer between triglyceride-rich lipoproteins and low density lipoproteins (LDLs) can raise HDL-cholesterol levels much more substantially than existing agents. What will be needed as these chemical agents are moved towards clinical use in humans is demonstration of their long-term safety and clear evidence in randomised controlled trials (RCTs) of efficacy in reducing disease burden.

12.2 What new lipid lowering drugs are in the pipeline?

STATINS IN THE FUTURE

The statins have been a major breakthrough in medical treatments, not just in their cholesterol and LDL-cholesterol lowering ability, but because they have made a major impact on coronary and cerebrovascular disease prevention. They have done this with a very low side effect rate, and are one of the very few groups of drugs to make a substantial impact on human longevity, and on good-quality longevity. As such they are not likely to be displaced as a major treatment in the foreseeable future. Other members of the class may come to market, such as pitavastatin, offering LDL-lowering ability of somewhat the same degree as atorvastatin and rosuvastatin.

However, after a potential reduction of cardiovascular disease (CVD) of around 30% to perhaps 50% at most, coupled with the benefits of aspirin and other agents, we will still be left with half or more of our patients suffering CVD. Other steps are going to be needed here.

HDL ADMINISTRATION

Of great interest was the result of experiments infusing high density lipoproteins. This was done using a synthesised HDL variant – HDL Milano – and demonstrated rapid beneficial changes in atheromatous arterial walls.

ELEVATION OF HDL-CHOLESTEROL

Epidemiologically, higher levels of HDL-cholesterol are protective for cardiovascular disease. This does not necessarily mean that all methods to elevate HDL will be beneficial. HDL levels could rise either because there is increased synthesis or if there is reduced clearance. HDL particles that may occur may not all have the same anti-atherogenic potential, and clearly the quality of HDLs is altered and likely to be less protective when triglycerides are high, for then there are triglyceride-rich particles.

In this area, however, modulation of cholesterol ester transfer protein (CETP; *see* Q 1.13) will shortly be possible with the first of a new class of inhibitors of this enzyme, torcetrapib. In hypertriglyceridaemic states the triglyceride-rich lipoproteins (in excess in the plasma) have a longer residence time in the plasma, and with upregulated CETP lead to triglyceride being exchanged into LDL and HDL with removal of cholesterol from LDL and HDL. This results in small dense LDL particles which are less readily removed by the classical Brown and Goldstein pathway, and which are more avidly taken up by the macrophage scavenger pathway in the arterial wall, the macrophage becoming the foam cell of the atherosclerotic fatty plaque. Similarly, alterations in the HDL particles occur which reduce in number and are less protective.

While complete inhibition of CETP may well be harmful, partial inhibition limits these changes and considerably (perhaps 40%) increases HDL quantity and protects its quality.

> Use of the inhibitor, torcetrapib, may therefore have a role in limiting atherogenesis, but longer term RCTs against hard endpoints of CVD rates will be needed. Use of torcetrapib will be in the context of an addition to current best practice (of statin used to lower LDL-cholesterol to new targets; <2 mmol/L) in patients at high risk with residual mixed hyperlipidaemia. For this reason, and also for commercial reasons, torcetrapib in a fixed dose will only be available in conjunction with variable doses of atorvastatin.

MIXED LIPAEMIA AND THE METABOLIC SYNDROME

We have a growing epidemic of obesity, associated with reduced exercise and maintained or increased calorie intake. This is leading to CVD, associated with insulin resistance and the metabolic syndrome (*see Q 4.3*). Metabolic syndrome has various definitions, but that of the USA Adult Treatment Panel Third Report (NCEP ATP-III)[1] is most often used. The diagnosis is made if at least three of the following are present:

1. waist circumference >40 inches (>102 cm) in males or >35 inches (>88 cm) in females
2. serum triglycerides: ≥1.7 mmol/L
3. HDL-cholesterol: <1.0 mmol/L in males or <1.3 mmol/L in females
4. blood pressure: ≥130/≥85 mmHg
5. fasting glucose: ≥6.1 mmol/L.

These patients will also have hypertriglyceridaemia and low HDL values as part of their dyslipidaemia, which will be contributing to their CVD risk through the generation of excess and atherogenic small dense LDLs together with abnormal HDLs. Here we will wish to see fibrates used, but will await the result of the FIELD study from Australia, and also a fibrate–statin combination outcome study.

INSULIN SENSITIVITY

What other treatments are we likely to see in our metabolic syndrome, insulin-resistant patients? Clearly, insulin sensitisers have a role in the treatment of diabetic patients, and may have a role currently under investigation to limit progression to diabetes in those at high risk (impaired glucose tolerant and impaired fasting glycaemic patients). Furthermore, if they do this, and if insulin resistance is pathogenic in macrovascular disease we may see positive results of the trials with thiazolidinediones to limit CVD.

The thiazolidinediones (the glitazones) modify cell receptors called peroxisome proliferator-activated receptors (PPARs), but these receptors also lead to adipogenesis, so the current glitazones are associated with some weight increase, albeit that the weight increase is associated with a beneficial movement of fat from visceral to subcutaneous stores. Newer glitazones without this type of effect would be advantageous, so-called SPPARMs – selective PPAR modulators.

CANNABINOID RECEPTOR INHIBITORS

Various weight-reducing drugs are available and will prevent progression to diabetes (orlistat). With weight loss come associated improvements in glucose, lipids and blood pressure.

A newer class of drug in development are the endo-cannabinoid receptor blockers. Rimonobant, the first of these in development by Sanofi-Aventis, has been shown to have significant weight-reducing effects with 58% of patients on 20 mg losing and maintaining the loss of >10% of body weight at 1 year, while improving HDL, lowering triglycerides and improving insulin sensitivity. Further studies showed patients could stop smoking without weight gain.

12.3 Is gene therapy a realistic possibility?

Gene therapy may become a possibility in the future for some dyslipidaemias. Studies of gene transfers and gene knockouts in animals have been able to demonstrate the effects that result, and allow some extrapolation to potential in man. Modulation of some pathways by gene treatments may not be appropriate, such as where many metabolic pathways are simultaneously modified. An example might be modulation of the PPAR system as multiple tissues and enzymes are up- or downregulated.

Familial hypercholesterolaemia (*see Q 4.6*) is clearly a very attractive single gene disorder where replacement of the gene for the LDL receptor into the liver would very substantially correct the disorder. While all tissues will be LDL receptor deficient, it is the liver that largely controls the circulating plasma LDL level. That there are many hundreds of different defects in the LDL receptor would not alter the issue, but to date gene treatment of familial hypercholesterolaemia is not on the near horizon.

A different situation is present for the very rare inherited condition of lipoprotein lipase (LPL) deficiency, which occurs in one in a million individuals. The LPL gene has been synthesised, and initial animal experiments have been successful. The potential for this to be extended to humans is imminent, but initially is likely to be limited to LPL-deficient individuals who have had severe and/or recurrent acute pancreatitis as this condition has substantial morbidity and mortality.

12.4 What are the important scientific issues to be settled by ongoing clinical trials?

In lipid and lipoprotein disorders, the most important issues relate to:

■ the optimal level of LDL-cholesterol
■ confirmation of the hypothesis that additional LDL lowering is valuable
■ the roles and outcomes for fibrates
■ whether pharmacological elevations of HDL are beneficial
■ whether modification of inflammatory markers and cytokines will influence atherogenesis and whether this is independent of or at least in part secondary to LDL-cholesterol lowering
■ whether improving insulin sensitivity will protect against atherosclerosis independently of lipids, blood pressure and glycated haemoglobin.

The recent lipid RCTs have demonstrated that there is the same relative risk reduction whether initial LDL levels are higher or lower, and that there is benefit to achieved LDL-cholesterol below 2 mmol/L.

The PROVE-IT study[2] demonstrated an additional 16% CVD benefit by lowering LDL-cholesterol by an additional 16% (using atorvastatin 80 mg compared to pravastatin 40 mg daily), fitting well with the general in-trial benefits of a 1% fall in LDL equating to around a 1% CVD fall. While this study compared two different statins, the presumption is that it is the LDL change that is responsible. This hypothesis is based on data from studies lasting 3–6 years, and in lifetime epidemiological data a 1% LDL change would reduce CVD by 2%. The A-to-Z study comparing 20 mg and 80 mg simvastatin (a potential 10–12% LDL difference) was more equivocal.[3] In TNT[4], comparing 10 mg and 80 mg atorvastatin, there were significant benefits of the higher dose. Two other studies comparing different statin doses – SEARCH and IDEAL – should report in 1–2 years' time.

There is considerable interest in high-sensitivity C-reactive protein (CRP) levels, which are elevated in individuals at increased CVD risk. CRP levels fall with statins, but quickly, and it is uncertain whether these are a consequence of LDL-cholesterol changes or due to non-lipid direct effects. Studies are being set up to look at this in more detail, and also in individuals who would be at quite low risk if it were not for the presence of elevated CRP.

As insulin resistance syndrome and metabolic syndrome patients have such high CVD risk, there is substantial research interest in understanding the roles and mechanisms involved. Some evidence suggests that metformin may reduce CVD risk. Major double-blind RCTs are currently in progress examining the potential benefits of the insulin sensitisers, the thiazolidinediones (the 'glitazones'), and data should be available in about 2 years.

A major study (called FIELD) of fenofibrate in mixed lipaemia patients is underway to determine if there is atheroprotection, and will report in about 2006. This study will have seen substantial co-prescribing of statins in this patient group, but it is hoped that it will still allow a definitive answer for fenofibrate. In the USA another study is recruiting, looking at fibrate and/or statin.

When torcetrapib comes to clinical use in the next 2–3 years a major question to be answered will be long-term hard endpoints for CVD. At present it is likely that torcetrapib will be available only in a combined preparation with atorvastatin. It is hoped that appropriate double-blind studies will take place using atorvastatin, together with torcetrapib or placebo.

12.5 What features of clinical guidelines are most likely to change?

Major changes are currently taking place in the clinical guidelines being put forward nationally and internationally. These are based on the widening evidence base for treatment benefit, and a number of changes will occur.

While the relationship between rising cholesterol and stroke is much flatter than that with coronary heart disease (CHD), the statin trials have demonstrated very significant reductions in stroke, greater than would be expected. Thus the term 'secondary prevention' is no longer confined to individuals with CHD, and all individuals with any atherosclerotic disease should be so treated, including those with peripheral arterial disease. There are some data accumulating to suggest that statins may also slow the progression of aortic stenosis.

It is now well recognised that individuals without CVD but with diabetes have such major increases in CVD risk that their disease rates often equate to those non-diabetic individuals who have overt CVD. The outcome data for type 2 diabetes are now extremely strong (CARDS,[5] HPS,[6] 4S[7]). While the number of individuals with type 1 diabetes in statin studies have been very small, it is very unlikely that a major RCT in this group will be possible. Patients who have had type 1 diabetes for over a decade or two (or more) have very high CVD rates, and the view is emerging that many of these individuals should be treated early. A further group of high risk individuals are those with significant renal disease and developing chronic renal failure. All of these individuals are now deemed to be treated as 'secondary' and not 'primary' prevention.

Following the Heart Protection Study,[6] where 5000 individuals with initial total cholesterol levels between 3.5 and 5.0 mmol/L showed similar relative CVD reductions as those with higher levels, the threshold for intervention in individuals at sufficient CVD risk will be a cholesterol >3.5 mmol/L.

Having decided that an individual has a sufficiently high global CVD risk, then all applicable risk factors will need to be tackled, and the targets for cholesterol and LDL-cholesterol will now be <4 mmol/L and <2 mmol/L, respectively. For non-HDL-cholesterol and for triglycerides, desirable values will be <3 mmol/L and <1.7 mmol/L, respectively. While these are desirable values, it will have to be recognised that not all individuals will be able to reach them, and this may have to suffice. Much benefit results from the initial treatments and lipid reductions. However, where possible the lower reductions should be achieved.

'Starter' doses of statins (or other agents) may be sufficient for many, but for some up-titration of treatment will be needed. The UK guidelines have already been set at the above levels, the previous European 2003 guidelines had set a <2.5 mmol/L target, while the recent revision of the NCEP ATP-III guidelines[1] have indicated that a target of <1.8 mmol/L may be appropriate for highest risk individuals.

In subsequent years there may be moves away from LDL- and HDL-cholesterol to use the specific apolipoproteins, apo-B and apo-AI (*see Q 1.8*), as indicators of risk and perhaps targets for treatment. Similarly, there may be developing intervention levels and targets for inflammatory markers such as hs-CRP. At present, the definitive data for such changes are not available.

APPENDIX
Useful organisations and websites

GP and patient information

Association of British Clinical Diabetologists (ABCD)
Dr P Wincour (Honorary Secretary)
Queen Elizabeth 2 Hospital
Howlands
Welwyn Garden City AL7 4HQ
Tel: 01707 365093
www.diabetologists.org.uk
   ABCD is the professional association for hospital consultants specialising in diabetes, with the aim of improving primary and secondary integrated diabetes care for NHS patients.

Blood Pressure Association
60 Cranmer Terrace
London SW17 0QS
Tel: 020 8772 4994
Fax: 020 8772 4999
www.bpassoc.org.uk
   The Association's aims are to draw attention to the need to improve detection, management and treatment of people with high blood pressure.

British Cardiac Patients Association
2 Station Road
Swavesey
Cambridge CB4 5QJ
Tel/fax: 01954 202022
Email: enquries@BCPA.co.uk
www.bcpa.co.uk
   Offers unconditional help, support, reassurance and advice to cardiac patients, their families and carers.

British Cardiac Society
9 Fitzroy Square
London W1T 5HW
Tel: 020 7383 3887
Fax: 020 7388 0903
www.bcs.com

The Society is involved in education, the setting of clinical standards and research into heart and circulatory diseases.

British Heart Foundation
14 Fitzhardinge Street
London W1H 6DH
Tel: 020 7935 0185
Fax: 020 7486 5820
Email: internet@bhf.org.uk
    Heart Information Line: 08450 70 80 70 (available Mon–Fri 9am–5pm, a free service for those seeking information on heart health issues)
www.bhf.org.uk
    The aim of the British Heart Foundation (BHF) is to play a leading role in the fight against heart disease so that it is no longer a major cause of disability and premature death by funding research into the causes, prevention, diagnosis and treatment of heart disease; providing support and information to heart patients and their families through BHF nurses, rehabilitation programmes and support groups; educating the public and health professionals about heart disease, its prevention and treatment; promoting training in emergency life support skills for the public and health professionals, and by providing vital life-saving equipment to hospitals and other health providers.

British Hypertension Society
Blood Pressure Unit, Department of Physiological Medicine
St George's Hospital Medical School
Cranmer Terrace
London SW17 0RE
Tel: 012 8725 3412
Fax: 020 8725 2959
Email: bhsis@sghms.ac.uk
www.hyp.ac.uk/bhs
    The BHS Information Service provides information about hypertension to doctors, nurses and other healthcare professionals, including hypertension management guidelines, validated blood pressure monitors, recommendations for combining antihypertensive drugs and blood pressure measurement recommendations.

Diabetes UK
10 Parkway
London NW1 7AA
Tel: 020 7424 1819
Fax: 020 7424 1001

E-mail: info@diabetes.org.uk
www.diabetes.org.uk

Diabetes UK is a charity working for people with diabetes. Its aim is to improve the lives of people with diabetes and to work towards a future without this serious condition.

HEART UK
7 North Road
Maidenhead
Berkshire SL6 1PE
Tel: 01628 628 638
Fax: 01628 628 698
Email: ask@heartuk.org.uk
www.heartuk.org.uk

HEART UK is the Hyperlipidaemia Education And Research Trust, formed from the British Hyperlipidaemia Association and the Family Heart Association. HEART UK provides information for patients and families with high cholesterol, and those at high risk of heart attack and stroke. HEART UK supports the need for scientific research and good clinical practice for the management of high blood cholesterol and blood fats in the UK.

National Obesity Forum (NOF)
PO Box 6625
Nottingham NG2 5PA
Tel/fax: 0115 8462109
www.nationalobesityforum.org.uk

The NOF was established in May 2000 to raise awareness of the growing impact of obesity and overweight on patients and professionals in the UK. Membership is open to all healthcare professionals and is free.

Primary Care Cardiovascular Society
36 Berrymede Road
London W4 5JD
Tel: 020 8994 8775
Fax: 020 8742 2130
Email: office@pccs.org.uk
www.pccs.org.uk

The aims of the PCCS are to improve the care and outcome of patients with cardiovascular disease through the exchange of knowledge, and the promotion amongst clinical practitioners of research, education and development relating to cardiovascular disease in general, and community cardiovascular medicine in particular.

Royal College of Physicians
11 St Andrews Place
Regent's Park
London NW1 4LE
Tel: 020 7935 1174
Fax: 020 7487 5218
www.rcplondon.ac.uk

The RCP aims to ensure high quality care for patients by improving standards and influencing policy and practice in modern medicine. It sets standards for clinical practice, conducts examinations, defines and monitors education and training programmes.

Government sites and guidelines

- **Clinical Resource Efficiency Support Team** (CREST), Northern Ireland www.crestni.org.uk
- **Health Development Agency** (publications, including patient information sheets on heart disease, in Gujerati, Bengali, Hindi and Punjabi) www.hda-online.org.uk
- **Health Survey for England** www.dh.gov.uk/PublicationsAndStatistics/ PublishedSurvey/HealthSurveyForEngland/fs/en
- **National Heart, Lung & Blood Institute** (United States). Direct links to: (1) guide to lowering high blood pressure: www.nhlbi.nih.gov/hbp/index.html; (2) National Cholesterol Education Program (NCEP): www.nhlbi.nih.gov/about/ncep
- **National Institute for Clinical Excellence** www.nice.org.uk
- **New GMS contract 2003** Quality indicators - summary of points. Secondary prevention in coronary heart disease www.bma.org.uk
- **Scottish Intercollegiate Guidelines Network** (SIGN) www.sign.ac.uk
- **UK National Service Framework for Coronary Heart Disease (2000)** www.nelh.nhs/uk/nsf/chd/nsf
- **UK National Service Framework for Diabetes (2000)** www.dh.gov.uk/PolicyAndGuidance/HealthAndSocialCareTopics/ Diabetes/fs/en
- **Welsh Assembly** (responsible for most of the issues of day-to-day concern to the people of Wales, including health and drug treatment) www.wales.gov.uk

Research

- **Canadian Cardiovascular Society** (journal-like website with information about cardiovascular research and resources in Canada) www.ccs.ca
- **Cardiac Society of Australia and New Zealand** www.csanz.edu.au

- **CORDA** (The Coronary Artery Disease Research Association) www.corda.org.uk
- **National Heart Research Fund** www.heartresearch.org.uk
- **US National Institutes of Health** (biomedical research, free) www.nih.gov/health

Informative websites for the GP and patient

- **American College of Cardiology** (professional website providing a framework of evidence-based clinical statements and guidelines) www.acc.org
- **American Dietetic Association** (public service promoting optimal nutrition, health and wellbeing) www.eatright.org
- **American Heart Association** (provides download patient information sheets that address cardiovascular conditions, treatments and tests, and lifestyle/risk reduction) www.americanheart.org
- **BHF National Centre for Physical Activity and Health** (develops and promotes initiatives to help professionals stimulate more people to take more activity as part of everyday life) www.bhfactive.org.uk
- **British Nutrition Foundation** www.nutrition.org.uk
- **European Atherosclerosis Society** (professional organisation devoted to advancing knowledge of the causes, natural history, treatment and prevention of atherosclerosis, including development of guidelines for the treatment and especially the prevention of atherosclerotic disease) www.eas-society.org
- **European Society of Cardiology (ESC)** (international society whose comprehensive website provides quick access links to guidelines and recommendations, distance learning, decision-making tools, ESC journals and educational products) www.escardio.org
- **HeartCenterOnline** (Online website for cardiologists and their patients. Links to advice on cholesterol via their Cholesterol Center subdivision) www.heartcenteronline.com
- **Heart Foundation** (Australia) www.heartfoundation.com.au
- **Heart Information Network** (US information website for patients) www.heartinfo.com
- **International Atherosclerosis Society (IAS)** (promotes the advancement of science, research and teaching in the field of atherosclerosis and related diseases) www.athero.org
- **International Society for the Study of Fatty Acids and Lipids** (aims to increase understanding through research and education of the role of dietary fatty acids and lipids in health and disease) www.issfal.org.uk
- **Lifeclinic** (patient website with links to blood pressure, diabetes, cholesterol and nutrition) www.lifeclinic.com

- **LipidDisorders** (a service of lipidhealth.org (www.lipidhealth.org) and the National Lipid Education Council as a gateway of information for healthcare professionals on the subject of statins) www.LipidDisorders.org
- **LipidsOnline** (online resource for clinicians, researchers and educators with an interest in atherosclerosis, dyslipidemia and lipid management) www.lipidsonline.org
- **Medicine Net** (US website with patient information on common conditions, including high blood pressure) www.focusonhighbloodpressure.com
- **Men's Health Forum** (addresses issues affecting the health and wellbeing of boys and men in England and Wales) www.menshealthforum.org.uk; see also sister website: www.malehealth.co.uk
- **Net Doctor** (UK patient information site) www.netdoctor.co.uk

Journals
- Direct links are provided by www.cardiosource.com/library/journals to: *American Heart Journal; American Journal of Cardiology; American Journal of Hypertension; Atherosclerosis; Evidence-Based Cardiovascular Medicine; International Journal of Cardiology; Journal of the American College of Cardiology; Lancet; Progess in Cardiovascular Diseases; Thrombosis Research; Trends in Cardiovascular Medicine*
- *American Journal of Clinical Nutrition* http://intl.ajcn.org
- *British Journal of Cardiology* www.bjcardio.co.uk
- *British Medical Journal* http://bmj.bmjjournals.com/cgi/collection/heart_failure
- *Circulation* http://circ.ahajournals.org (also provides direct links to the following journals: *Arteriosclerosis, Thrombosis and Vascular Biology, Circulation Research, Hypertension, Stroke*)
- *Current Opinion in Lipidology* www.co-lipidology.com
- *Drugs in Context* www.drugsincontext.com (the publishers of this journal – CSF Medical Communications – have also published a book for patients in their BESTMEDICINE series, entitled *Lipid Disorders* – see www.csfmedical.com/bestmedicine.asp)
- *European Heart Journal* www.eurheartj.org
- *Heart* http://heart.bmjjournals.com
- *Journal of the American Medical Association* http://jama.ama-assn.org
- *Journal of Atherosclerosis and Thrombosis* http://jas.umin.ac.jp/en/joaat.html
- *Journal of Lipid Research* www.jlr.org
- *Lipids in Health and Disease* www.lipidworld.com
- *National Electronic Library for Health* (Specialist Library for Cardiovascular Diseases) http://rms.nelh.nhs.uk/cardiovascular
- *New England Journal of Medicine* www.nejm.org

REFERENCES

CHAPTER 1

1. Chen Z, Peto R, Collins R et al 1991 Serum cholesterol concentration and coronary heart disease in a population with low cholesterol concentrations. BMJ 303:276–282
2. Expert Panel on Detection, Evaluation and Treatment of High Blood Cholesterol in Adults 2001 Executive Summary of the Third Report of the National Cholesterol Education Program (NCEP) Expert Panel on Detection, Evaluation and Treatment of High Blood Cholesterol in Adults (Adult Treatment Panel III). JAMA 285:2486–2497

CHAPTER 2

1. Chen Z, Peto R, Collins R et al 1991 Serum cholesterol concentration and coronary heart disease in a population with low cholesterol concentrations. BMJ 303:276–282
2. Keys A, Anderson JT, Grande F 1958 Lessons from serum cholesterol studies in Japan, Hawaii and Los Angeles. Ann Intern Med 48:83–94
3. Ross R 1993 The pathogenesis of atherosclerosis: a perspective for the 1990s. Nature 362(6423):801–809
4. Verschuren WM, Jacobs DR, Bloemberg BP et al 1995 Serum total cholesterol and long-term coronary heart disease mortality in different cultures. Twenty-five-year follow-up of the seven countries study. JAMA 274(2):131–136
5. Castelli WP 1984 Epidemiology of coronary heart disease: the Framingham study. Am J Med 76(2A):4–12

6. Neaton JD, Kuller L, Wentworth D et al 1984 Total and cardiovascular mortality in relation to cigarette smoking, serum cholesterol concentration, and diastolic blood pressure among black and white males followed up for 5 years. Am Heart J 108:759–769
7. Stamler J, Wentworth D, Neaton JD for the MRFIT Research Group 1986 Is relationship between serum cholesterol and risk of premature death from coronary heart disease continuous and graded? Findings in 356,222 primary screenees of the Multiple Risk Factor Intervention Trial (MRFIT). JAMA 256:2823–2828
8. Stamler J, Stamler R, Neaton JD 1993 Blood pressure, systolic and diastolic, and cardiovascular risks. US population data. Arch Intern Med 153(5):598–615
9. British Cardiac Society, British Hypertension Society, Diabetes UK, HEART UK, Primary Care Cardiovascular Society, Stroke Association 2005 Joint British Societies' guidelines-2 (JBS-2) for the primary prevention of cardiovascular disease in clinical practice. Heart (in press)
10. Heart Protection Study Collaborative Group 2002 MRC/BHF Heart Protection Study of cholesterol lowering with simvastatin in 20,536 high-risk individuals: a randomised placebo-controlled trial. Lancet 360:7–22
11. Sever PS, Dahlof B, Poulter NR et al for the ASCOT investigators 2004 Prevention of coronary and stroke events with atorvastatin in

hypertensive patients who have average or lower than average cholesterol concentrations, in the Anglo-Scandinavian Cardiac Outcomes Trial – Lipid Lowering Arm (ASCOT-LLA): a multicentre randomised controlled trial. Lancet 361:1149–1158

12. Athyros VG, Papageorgiou AA, Mercouris BR 2002 The GREek Atorvastatin and Coronary heart disease Evaluation (GREACE) study. Curr Med Res Opin 18:220–228

13. Serruys PW, de Feyter P, Macaya C et al; Lescol Intervention Prevention Study (LIPS) investigators 2002 Fluvastatin for prevention of cardiac events following successful first percutaneous coronary intervention: a randomised controlled trial. JAMA 287:3215–3222

14. Colhoun HM, Betteridge DJ, Durrington PN et al 2004 Primary prevention of cardiovascular disease with atorvastatin in type 2 diabetes in the Collaborative Atorvastatin Diabetes Study (CARDS): multicentre randomised placebo-controlled trial. Lancet 364:685–696

15. Cannon CP, Braunwald E, McCabe CH et al 2004 Pravastatin or atorvastatin evaluation and infection therapy – Thrombolysis In Myocardial Infarction 22 (TIMI-22) investigators. Intensive versus moderate lipid lowering with statins after acute coronary syndromes. N Engl J Med 350:1495–1504

16. LaRosa JC, Grundy SM, Waters DD et al, for the Treating to New Targets (TNT) Investigators 2005 Intensive lipid lowering with atorvastatin in patients with stable coronary disease. N Engl J Med 352:1425–1435

17. Keys A (ed) 1970 Coronary heart disease in seven countries. Circulation 40 (Suppl 1):I-186–I-198

18. Expert Panel on Detection, Evaluation and Treatment of High Blood Cholesterol in Adults 2001 Executive Summary of the Third Report of the National Cholesterol Education Program (NCEP) Expert Panel on Detection, Evaluation and Treatment of High Blood Cholesterol in Adults (Adult Treatment Panel III). JAMA 285:2486–2497

CHAPTER 3

1. Expert Panel on Detection, Evaluation and Treatment of High Blood Cholesterol in Adults 2001 Executive Summary of the Third Report of the National Cholesterol Education Program (NCEP) Expert Panel on Detection, Evaluation and Treatment of High Blood Cholesterol in Adults (Adult Treatment Panel III). JAMA 285:2486–2497

2. Sniderman AD, Furberg CD, Keech A et al 2003 Apolipoproteins versus lipids as indices of coronary risk and as targets for statin treatment. Lancet 361:777–780

3. Friedewald WT, Levy R, Frederickson DS 1972 Estimation of the concentration of low density lipoprotein cholesterol in plasma without the use of the preparative ultracentrifuge. Clin Chem 18:499–502

4. Beaumont JL, Carlson LA, Cooper GR et al 1970 Classification of hyper-lipidaemia and hyperlipoproteinaemia. Bull WHO 43:891–915

5. Durrington P 2003 Dyslipidaemia. Lancet 362:717–731

6. Kannel WB 1988 Nutrition and the occurrence and prevention of cardiovascular disease in the elderly. Nutr Rev 46:66–78

CHAPTER 4

1. Expert Panel on Detection, Evaluation and Treatment of High Blood

Cholesterol in Adults 2001 Executive Summary of the Third Report of the National Cholesterol Education Program (NCEP) Expert Panel on Detection, Evaluation and Treatment of High Blood Cholesterol in Adults (Adult Treatment Panel III). JAMA 285:2486–2497

CHAPTER 5

1. British Cardiac Society, British Hypertension Society, Diabetes UK, HEART UK, Primary Care Cardio-vascular Society, Stroke Association 2005 Joint British Societies' guidelines-2 (JBS-2) for the primary prevention of cardiovascular disease in clinical practice. Heart (in press)

2. Expert Panel on Detection, Evaluation and Treatment of High Blood Cholesterol in Adults 2001 Executive Summary of the Third Report of the National Cholesterol Education Program (NCEP) Expert Panel on Detection, Evaluation and Treatment of High Blood Cholesterol in Adults (Adult Treatment Panel III). JAMA 285:2486–2497

3. De Backer G, Ambrosioni E, Borch-Johnsen K et al 2003 European guidelines on cardiovascular disease prevention in clinical practice: Third Joint Task Force of European and other Societies on Cardiovascular Disease Prevention in Clinical Practice. Eur Heart J 24:1601–1610

4. Conroy RM, Pyörälä K, Fitzgerald AP et al 2003 Estimation of ten-year risk of fatal cardiovascular disease in Europe: the SCORE project. Eur Heart J 24:987–1003

5. Grover SA, Coupal I, Xiao-Ping H et al 1995 Identifying adults at increased risk of coronary heart disease. How well do the current cholesterol guidelines work? JAMA 274:801–806

6. Brindle P, Emberson J, Lampe F et al 2003 Predictive accuracy of the Framingham coronary risk score in British men: prospective cohort study. BMJ 327:1267–1270

7. Yusuf S, Hawken S, Ounpuu S et al 2004 Effect of potentially modifiable risk factors associated with myocardial infarction in 52 countries (the INTERHEART study): case-control study. Lancet 364:937–952

8. Haq IU, Ramsay LE, Wallis EJ et al 2001 Population implications of lipid lowering for the prevention of coronary heart disease: data from the 1995 Scottish Health Survey. Heart 86:289–295

9. Cappucio F, Oakeshott P, Strazullo P et al 2002 Application of Framingham risk estimates to ethnic minorities in United Kingdom and implications for primary prevention of heart disease in general practice: cross sectional population based study. BMJ 325:1271–1274

CHAPTER 6

1. DiClemente C, Prochaska J, Fairhurst SK et al 1991 The process of smoking cessation: an analysis of precontemplation, contemplation and preparation stages of change. J Consult Clin Psychol 59:295–304

2. Ornish D, Brown S, Scherwitz LW et al 1990 Can lifestyle changes reverse coronary heart disease? The Lifestyle Heart Trial. Lancet 336:129–133

3. Neil H, Hawkins M, Durrington P et al for the Simon Broome Familial Hyperlipidaemia Register Group and Scientific Steering Committee 2005 Non-coronary heart disease mortality and risk of fatal cancer in patients with treated heterozygous familial hypercholesterolaemia: a prospective registry study. Atherosclerosis 179:293–297

4. Garrow JS 1981 Treat obesity seriously. Edinburgh: Churchill Livingstone

5. Després J-P, Lemieux I, Prud'homme D 2001 Treatment of obesity: need to focus on high risk abdominally obese patients. BMJ 322:716–720

6. Dattilo AM, Kris-Etherton PM 1992 Effects of weight reduction on blood lipids and lipoproteins: a meta-analysis. Am J Clin Nutr 56:320–328

7. Hooper L, Summerbell CD, Higgins JPT et al 2001 Dietary fat intake and prevention of cardiovascular disease: systematic review. BMJ 322:757–763

8. Tang JL, Armitage JM, Lancaster T et al 1998 Systematic review of dietary intervention trials to lower blood cholesterol in free-living subjects. BMJ 316:1213–1220

9. Jula A, Marniemi J, Huupponen R et al 2002 Effects of diet and simvastatin on serum lipids, insulin, and antioxidants in hypercholesterolemic men: a randomized controlled trial. JAMA 287:598–605

10. De Lorgeril M, Salen P, Martin JL et al 1999 Mediterranean diet, traditional risk factors and the rate of cardiovascular complications after myocardial infarction: the final report of the Lyon Diet Heart Study. Circulation 99:779–785

11. American Heart Association 2000 AHA dietary guidelines: revision 2000. Circulation 102:2284–2299

12. Burr ML, Fehily AM, Gilbert JF et al 1989 Effects of changes in fat, fish and fiber intakes on death and myocardial reinfarction trial (DART). Lancet 2:757–761

13. GISSI-Prevenzione Investigators 1999 Dietary supplementation with n-3 polyunsaturated fatty acids and vitamin E after myocardial infarction: results of the GISSI-Prevenzione Trial. Lancet 354:447–455

14. Katan MB, Grundy SM, Jones P et al 2003 Efficacy and safety of plant stanols and sterols in the management of blood cholesterol levels. Mayo Clin Proc 78:965–978

15. Erdman JW 2000 Soy protein and cardiovascular disease. Circulation 102:2555–2559

16. Brown L, Rosner B, Willett W et al 1999 Cholesterol-lowering effects of dietary fiber: a meta-analysis. Am J Clin Nutr 69:30–42

17. Jenkins DJA, Kendall CWC, Faulkner D et al 2002 A dietary portfolio approach to cholesterol reduction: combined effects of plant sterols, vegetable proteins, and viscous fibers in hypercholesterolaemia. Metabolism 51:1596–1604

18. Jenkins DJ, Kendal CW, Marchie A et al 2003 Effects of a dietary portfolio of cholesterol-lowering foods vs lovastation on serum lipids and C-reactive protein. JAMA 290:502–510

19. Foster GD, Wyatt HR, Hill JO et al 2003 A randomised trial of a low carbohydrate diet for obesity. N Engl J Med 348:2082–2090

CHAPTER 7

1. Wood DA, Durrington P, Poulter N et al on behalf of British Cardiac Society, British Hyperlipidaemia Association, British Hypertension Society, British Diabetic Association 1998 Joint British recommendations on prevention of coronary heart disease in clinical practice. Heart 80:S1–S29

2. Ballantyne CM, Corsini A, Davidson MH et al 2003 Risk for myopathy with statin therapy in high-risk patients: expert panel review. Arch Intern Med 163:553–564

3. Holdaas H, Fellstrom B, Jardine AG et al 2003 Effect of fluvastatin on

cardiac outcomes in renal transplant recipients: a multicentre, randomised, placebo-controlled trial. Lancet 361(9374):2024–2031

4. Cannon CP, Braunwald E, McCabe CH et al 2004 Pravastatin or atorvastatin evaluation and infection therapy – Thrombolysis In Myocardial Infarction 22 (TIMI-22) investigators. Intensive versus moderate lipid lowering with statins after acute coronary syndromes. N Engl J Med 350:1495–1504

5. LaRosa JC, Grundy SM, Waters DD et al, for the Treating to New Targets (TNT) Investigators 2005 Intensive lipid lowering with atorvastatin in patients with stable coronary disease. N Engl J Med 352:1425–1435

6. Williams B, Poulter N, Brown MJ et al 2004 Guidelines for the management of hypertension: report of the fourth working party of the British Hypertension Society 2004 (BHS-IV). J Hum Hypertens 18:139–185

7. Williams B, Poulter NR, Brown MJ et al; BHS guidelines working party, for the British Hypertension Society 2004 British Hypertension Society guidelines for hypertension management 2004 (BHS-IV): summary. BMJ 328(7440):634–640 (illustrations not shown in the paper journal can be accessed online at: www.hyp.ac.uk/bhs/ Latest_BHS_management_Guidelines. htm)

8. British Cardiac Society, British Hypertension Society, Diabetes UK, HEART UK, Primary Care Cardiovascular Society, Stroke Association 2005 Joint British Societies' guidelines-2 (JBS-2) for the primary prevention of cardiovascular disease in clinical practice. Heart (in press)

9. Expert Panel on Detection, Evaluation and Treatment of High Blood Cholesterol in Adults 2001 Executive Summary of the Third Report of the National Cholesterol Education Program (NCEP) Expert Panel on Detection, Evaluation and Treatment of High Blood Cholesterol in Adults (Adult Treatment Panel III). JAMA 285:2486–2497

10 Grundy SM, Vega GL, Yuan Z et al 2005 Effectiveness and tolerability of simvastatin plus fenofibrate for combined hyperlipidemia (The SAFARI trial). Am J Cardiol 95:462–468

11. Frick MH, Elo O, Haapa K et al 1987 Helsinki Heart Study: primary prevention trial with gemfibrozil in middle-aged men with dyslipidaemia. N Engl J Med 317:1237–1245

12. Bloomfield Rubins H, Robins SJ, Collins D et al for the Veterans Affairs High-density Lipoprotein Cholesterol Intervention Trial Study Group 1999 Gemfibrozil for the secondary prevention of coronary heart disease in men with low levels of high density lipoprotein cholesterol. N Engl J Med 341:410–418

13. Farnier M, Freeman MW, Macdonell G et al 2005 Efficacy and safety of the coadministration of ezetimibe with fenofibrate in patients with mixed hyperlipidaemia. Eur Heart J Apr 4 [Epub ahead of print]

14. Ascherio A, Rimm EB, Stampfer JM et al 1995 Dietary intake of marine n-3 fatty acids, fish intake and risk of coronary heart disease among men. N Engl J Med 332:977–982

15. McCarron P, Greenwood R, Elwood P et al 2001 The incidence and aetiology of stroke in the Caerphilly and Speedwell Collaborative Studies II: risk factors for ischaemic stroke. Public Health 115:12–20

16. GISSI-Prevenzione Investigators 1999 Dietary supplementation with n-3 polyunsaturated fatty acids and vitamin E after myocardial infarction: results of the GISSI-Prevenzione Trial. Lancet 354:447–455

17. Lipid Research Clinics Program 1984 The Lipid Research Clinics Coronary Primary Prevention Trial (LRC-CPPT) results. I. Reduction in incidence of coronary heart disease. JAMA 251:351–364

18. Lipid Research Clinics Program 1984 The Lipid Research Clinics Coronary Primary Prevention Trial (LRC-CPPT) results. II. The relationship of reduction in incidence of coronary heart disease to cholesterol lowering. JAMA 251:365–374

19. Watts GF, Lewis B, Brunt JN et al 1992 Effects on coronary artery disease of lipid-lowering diet, or diet plus cholestyramine, in the St Thomas' Atherosclerosis Regression Study (STARS). Lancet 339(8793):563–569

20. Lawrence JM, Reid J, Taylor GJ et al 2004 Favourable effects of pioglitazone and metformin compared with gliclazide on lipoprotein subfractions in overweight patients with early type 2 diabetes. Diabetes Care 27:41–46

21. Mukhtar R, Reckless JPD 2005 Dyslipidaemia in type 2 diabetes: effects of the thiazolidinediones pioglitazone and rosiglitazone. Diabet Med (in press)

CHAPTER 8

1. Frick MH, Elo O, Haapa K et al 1987 Helsinki Heart Study: primary prevention trial with gemfibrozil in middle-aged men with dyslipidaemia. N Engl J Med 317:1237–1245

2. Lipid Research Clinics Program 1984 The Lipid Research Clinics Coronary Primary Prevention Trial (LRC-CPPT) results. I. Reduction in incidence of coronary heart disease. JAMA 251:351–364

3. Lipid Research Clinics Program 1984 The Lipid Research Clinics Coronary Primary Prevention Trial (LRC-CPPT) results. II. The relationship of reduction in incidence of coronary heart disease to cholesterol lowering. JAMA 251:365–374

4. Watts GF, Lewis B, Brunt JN et al 1992 Effects on coronary artery disease of lipid-lowering diet, or diet plus cholestyramine, in the St Thomas' Atherosclerosis Regression Study (STARS). Lancet 339(8793):563–569

5. Martin MJ, Hulley SB, Browner WS et al 1986 Serum cholesterol, blood pressure and mortality: implications from a cohort of 361,662 men. Lancet 2:933–936

6. Scandinavian Simvastatin Survival Study Group 1994 Randomised trial of cholesterol lowering in 4,444 patients with coronary heart disease: the Scandinavian Simvastatin Survival Study (4S). Lancet 344:1383–1389

7. Pyorala K, Pedersen TR, Kjekshus J et al 1997 Cholesterol lowering with simvastatin improves prognosis of diabetic patients with coronary heart disease: a subgroup analysis of the Scandinavian Simvastatin Survival Study (4S). Diabetes Care 20:614–620

8. The Cholesterol and Recurrent Events Trial Investigators 1996 The effect of pravastatin on coronary events after myocardial infarction in patients with average cholesterol levels. N Engl J Med 335:1001–1009

9. The Long-Term Intervention with Pravastatin in Ischaemic Disease (LIPID) Study Group 1998 Prevention of cardiovascular events and death with pravastatin in patients with coronary heart disease and a broad

range of initial cholesterol levels.
N Engl J Med 339:1349–1357

10. Goldberg RB, Mellies MJ, Sacks FM et al 1998 Cardiovascular events and their reduction with pravastatin in diabetic and glucose-intolerant myocardial infarction survivors with average cholesterol levels: subgroup analyses in the cholesterol and recurrent events (CARE) trial. Circulation 98:2513–2519

11. Serruys PW, de Feyter P, Macaya C et al; Intervention Prevention Study (LIPS) investigators 2002 Fluvastatin for prevention of cardiac events following successful first percutaneous coronary intervention: a randomised controlled trial. JAMA 287:3215–3222

12. Holdaas H, Fellstrom B, Jardine AG et al 2003 Effect of fluvastatin on cardiac outcomes in renal transplant recipients: a multicentre, randomised, placebo-controlled trial. Lancet 361(9374):2024–2031

13. Shepherd J, Cobbe SM, Ford I et al for the West of Scotland Coronary Prevention Study Group 1995 Prevention of coronary heart disease with pravastatin in men with hypercholesterolaemia. N Engl J Med 333:1301–1307

14. Down JR, Clearfield M, Weis S et al for the AFCAPS/TexCAPS Research Group 1998 Primary prevention of acute coronary events with lovastatin in men and women with average cholesterol levels: results of AFCAPS/TexCAPS. JAMA 279:1615–1622

15. Sever PS, Dahlof B, Poulter NR et al 2004 Prevention of coronary and stroke events with atorvastatin in hypertensive patients who have average or lower than average cholesterol concentrations, in the Anglo-Scandinavian Cardiac Outcomes Trial – Lipid Lowering Arm (ASCOT-LLA): a multicentre randomised controlled trial. Lancet 361:1149–1158

16. Colhoun HM, Betteridge DJ, Durrington PN et al 2004 Primary prevention of cardiovascular disease with atorvastatin in type 2 diabetes in the Collaborative Atorvastatin Diabetes Study (CARDS): multicentre randomised placebo-controlled trial. Lancet 364:685–696

17. Heart Protection Study Collaborative Group 2002 MRC/BHF Heart Protection Study of cholesterol lowering with simvastatin in 20,536 high-risk individuals: a randomised placebo-controlled trial. Lancet 360:7–22

18. Heart Protection Study Collaborative Group 2003 MRC/BHF Heart Protection Study of cholesterol lowering with simvastatin in 5,963 people with diabetes: a randomised placebo-controlled trial. Lancet 361: 2005–2016

19. Cannon CP, Braunwald E, McCabe CH et al 2004 Pravastatin or atorvastatin evaluation and infection therapy – Thrombolysis In Myocardial Infarction 22 (TIMI-22) investigators. Intensive versus moderate lipid lowering with statins after acute coronary syndromes. N Engl J Med 350:1495–1504

20. LaRosa JC, Grundy SM, Waters DD et al, for the Treating to New Targets (TNT) Investigators 2005 Intensive lipid lowering with atorvastatin in patients with stable coronary disease. N Engl J Med 352:1425–1435

21. Zhang X, Patel A, Horibe H et al 2003 Cholesterol, coronary heart disease, and stroke in the Asia Pacific region. Int J Epidemiol 32:563–572

22. British Cardiac Society, British Hypertension Society, Diabetes UK,

HEART UK, Primary Care Cardiovascular Society, Stroke Association 2005 Joint British Societies' guidelines-2 (JBS-2) for the primary prevention of cardiovascular disease in clinical practice. Heart (in press)

23. Grundy SM, Cleeman JI, Merz CNB et al for the Coordinating Committee of the National Cholesterol Education Program 2004 Implication of recent clinical trials for the National Cholesterol Education Program Adult Treatment Panel III guidelines. Circulation 109:3112–3121

CHAPTER 9

1. EUROASPIRE I and II Group 2001 Clinical reality of coronary prevention guidelines: a comparison of EUROASPIRE I and II in nine countries. Lancet 357:995–1001

2. De Lusignan S, Dzregah B, Hague N et al 2003 Cholesterol management in patients with IHD: an audit-based appraisal of progress towards clinical targets in primary care. Br J Cardiol 10:223–228

3. Pearson TA, Laurora I, Chu H et al 2000 The Lipid Treatment Assessment Project (L-TAP): a multicenter survey to evaluate the percentages of dyslipidaemic patients receiving lipid-lowering therapy and achieving low-density lipoprotein goals. Arch Intern Med 160:459–467

4. Murchie P, Campbell NC, Ritchie LD et al 2003 Secondary prevention clinics for coronary heart disease: four year follow up of a randomised controlled trial in primary care. BMJ 326:84–87

5. British Hypertension Society Guidelines Working Party 2004 British Hypertension Society guidelines for hypertension management 2004 (BHS-IV): summary. BMJ 328:634–640. Online. Available: www.bhsoc.org

6. British Cardiac Society, British Hypertension Society, Diabetes UK, HEART UK, Primary Care Cardiovascular Society, Stroke Association 2005 Joint British Societies' guidelines-2 (JBS-2) for the primary prevention of cardiovascular disease in clinical practice. Heart (in press)

7. De Backer G, Ambrosioni E, Borch-Johnsen K et al 2003 European guidelines on cardiovascular disease prevention in clinical practice: Third Joint Task Force of European and other Societies on Cardiovascular Disease Prevention in Clinical Practice. Eur Heart J 24:1601–1610

8. Expert Panel on Detection, Evaluation and Treatment of High Blood Cholesterol in Adults 2001 Executive Summary of the Third Report of the National Cholesterol Education Program (NCEP) Expert Panel on Detection, Evaluation and Treatment of High Blood Cholesterol in Adults (Adult Treatment Panel III). JAMA 285:2486–2497

9. Coordinating Committee of the National Cholesterol Education Program 2004 Implications of recent clinical trials for the National Cholesterol Education Program Adult Treatment Panel III Guidelines. Circulation 110:227–239

10. Brady AJB, Betteridge DJ 2003 Prevalence and risks of undertreatment with statins. Br J Cardiol 10:218–219

11. La Rosa JC, He J, Vupputuri S 1999 Effect of statins on risk of coronary disease: a meta-analysis of randomised controlled trials. JAMA 282:2340–2346

12. Anon 2001 Randomised trial of a perindopril-based blood-pressure-lowering regimen among 6,105 individuals with previous stroke or transient ischaemic attack. Lancet 358:1033–1041

13. Wald NJ, Law MR 2003 A strategy to reduce cardiovascular disease by more than 80%. BMJ 326:1419–1423

CHAPTER 10

1. Stein EA, Illingworth DR, Kwitorovich et al 1999 Efficacy and safety of lovastatin in adolescent males with heterozygous familial hypercholesterolaemia: a randomised controlled trial. JAMA 281:137–144
2. Wiegman A, Hutten B, de Groot E et al 2004 Efficacy and safety of statin therapy in children with familial hypercholesterolaemia. JAMA 292:331–337
3. Shepherd J, Blauw GJ, Murphy MB et al 2002 Pravastatin in elderly individuals at risk of vascular disease (PROSPER): a randomised controlled trial. Lancet 360:1623–1630
4. Manson JM, Freyssinges C, Ducrocq MB et al 1996 Postmarketing surveillance of lovastatin and simvastatin exposure during pregnancy. Reprod Toxicol 10(6):439–446
5. Edison RJ, Muenke M 2004 Central nervous system and limb anomalies in case reports of first-trimester statin exposure. N Engl J Med 350(15):1579–1582
6. Writing Group for the Women's Health Initiative Investigators 2002 Risks and benefits of estrogen plus progestin in healthy postmenopausal women: principal results from the Women's Health Initiative randomised controlled trial. JAMA 288:321–333
7. Williams B, Poulter N, Brown MJ et al 2004 Guidelines for the management of hypertension: report of the fourth working party of the British Hypertension Society 2004 (BHS-IV). J Hum Hypertens 18:139–185
8. American College of Cardiology (ACC) 2005 54th Annual Scientific Session. Late-Breaking Clinical Trials II. Online. Available:

www.acc.org/media/session_info/late/ACC05/lbct_tuesday.htm

9. The ALLHAT Officers and Coordinators for the ALLHAT Collaborative Research Group 2002 Major outcomes in moderately hypercholesterolaemic, hypertensive patients randomized to pravastatin vs usual care: the Antihypertensive and Lipid-lowering Treatment to Prevent Heart Attack Trial (ALLHAT-LLT). JAMA 288:2998–3007
10. Sever PS, Dahlöf P, Poulter NR et al 2003 Prevention of coronary and stroke events with atorvastatin in hypertensive patients who have average or lower-than-average cholesterol concentrations, in the Anglo-Scandinavian Cardiac Outcomes Trial – Lipid Lowering Arm (ASCOT-LLA): a multicentre controlled trial. Lancet 361:1149–1158
11. UK Prospective Diabetes Study (UKPDS) 1998 Effect of intensive blood glucose control with metformin on complications in overweight patients with type 2 diabetes (UKPDS 34). Lancet 352:854–865
12. Colhoun HM, Betteridge DJ, Durrington PN et al 2004 Primary prevention of cardiovascular disease with atorvastation in type 2 diabetes in the Collaborative Atorvastatin Diabetes Study (CARDS): multicentre randomised placebo-controlled trial. Lancet 364:685–696
13. Diabetes Atherosclerosis Intervention Study Investigators 2001 Effect of fenofibrate on progression of coronary artery disease in type 2 diabetes: the Diabetes Atherosclerosis Intervention Study, a randomised study. Lancet 357:905–910
14. Meade T, Zuhrie R, Cook C et al 2002 Bezafibrate in men with lower extremity arterial disease: randomised controlled trial. BMJ 325:1139

CHAPTER 11

1. Johannesson M, Jönsson B, Kjekhus J et al 1997 Cost effectiveness of simvastatin treatment to lower cholesterol levels in patients with coronary heart disease. N Engl J Med 336:332–336

2. Jönsson B, Johannesson M, Kjekhus J et al 1996 Cost-effectiveness of cholesterol lowering. Results from the Scandinavian Simvastatin Survival Study (4S). Eur Heart J 17:1001–1007

3. Caro J, Klittich W, McGuire A et al 1997 The West of Scotland coronary prevention study: economic benefit analysis of primary prevention with pravastatin. BMJ 315:1577–1582

4. Pickin DM, McCabe CJ, Ramsay LE et al 1999 Cost effectiveness of HMG-CoA reductase inhibitor (statin) treatment related to the risk of coronary heart disease and cost of drug treatment. Heart 82:325–332

CHAPTER 12

1. Expert Panel on Detection, Evaluation and Treatment of High Blood Cholesterol in Adults 2001 Executive Summary of the Third Report of the National Cholesterol Education Program (NCEP) Expert Panel on Detection, Evaluation and Treatment of High Blood Cholesterol in Adults (Adult Treatment Panel III). JAMA 285:2486–2497

2. Cannon CP, Braunwald E, McCabe CH et al 2004 Pravastatin or atorvastatin evaluation and infection therapy – Thrombolysis In Myocardial Infarction 22 (TIMI-22) investigators. Intensive versus moderate lipid lowering with statins after acute coronary syndromes. N Engl J Med 350:1495–1504

3. de Lemos JA, Blazing MA, Wiviott SD et al for the A to Z Investigators 2004 Early intensive vs a delayed conservative simvastatin strategy in patients with acute coronary syndromes: Phase Z of the A to Z Trial. JAMA 292(11):1307–1316

4. LaRosa JC, Grundy SM, Waters DD et al, for the Treating to New Targets (TNT) Investigators 2005 Intensive lipid lowering with atorvastatin in patients with stable coronary disease. N Engl J Med 352:1425–1435

5. Colhoun HM, Betteridge DJ, Durrington PN et al 2004 Primary prevention of cardiovascular disease with atorvastatin in type 2 diabetes in the Collaborative Atorvastatin Diabetes Study (CARDS): multicentre randomised placebo-controlled trial. Lancet 364:685–696

6. Heart Protection Study Collaborative Group 2002 MRC/BHF Heart Protection Study of cholesterol lowering with simvastatin in 20,536 high-risk individuals: a randomised placebo-controlled trial. Lancet 360:7–22

7. Pyorala K, Pedersen TR, Kjekshus J et al 1997 Cholesterol lowering with simvastatin improves prognosis of diabetic patients with coronary heart disease: a subgroup analysis of the Scandinavian Simvastatin Survival Study (4S). Diabetes Care 20:614–620

GLOSSARY OF ACRONYMS AND ABBREVIATIONS

4D – Die Deutsche Diabetes Dialyse [study]
4S – Scandinavian Simvastatin Survival Study
AFCAPS – Air Force Coronary Atherosclerosis Prevention Study
ALERT – Assessment of LEscol in Renal Transplantation [study]
ALLHAT – Antihypertensive and Lipid Lowering treatment to prevent Heart Attack Trial
ALP – atherogenic lipoprotein profile [or phenotype]
ALT – alanine aminotransferase
AMORIS – Apolipoprotein-related Mortality Risk [study]
apo-A – apolipoprotein-A
apo-B – apolipoprotein-B
ASCOT – Anglo-Scandinavian Cardiac Outcomes Trial
AST – aspartate aminotransferase
BIP – Bezafibrate Infarction Prevention [trial]
CARDS – Collaborative Atorvastatin Diabetes Study
CARE – Cholesterol and Recurrent Events [trial]
CETP – cholesterol ester transfer protein
CHD – coronary heart disease
CPK, CK – creatinine (phospho)kinase
CRP – C-reactive protein
CVD – cardiovascular disease
DAIS – Diabetes Atherosclerosis Intervention Study
DART – Diet and Reinfarction Trial
DHA – docosahexaenoic acid
ELITE – Evaluation of Losartan In The Elderly [study]
EPA – eicosapentaenoic acid
ERA – Estrogen Replacement and Atherosclerosis [trial]
FDB – familial defective apo-B100
FH – familial hypercholesterolaemia
FIELD – Fenofibrate Intervention and Event Lowering in Diabetes [study]
GMS – General Medical Services

GREACE – GREek Atorvastatin and Coronary heart disease Evaluation [study]
HAART – highly active antiretroviral therapy
HbA1c – haemoglobin A1c
HDL – high density lipoprotein
HERS – Heart and Estrogen/progestin Replacement Study
HHS – Helsinki Heart Study
HMG-CoA – 3-hydroxy-3-methylglutaryl coenzyme-A [reductase]
HPS – Heart Protection Study
IDEAL – Incremental Decrease in Endpoints through Aggressive Lipid lowering [trial]
IDL – intermediate density lipoprotein
LCAT – lecithin cholesterol acyl transferase
LDL – low density lipoprotein
LEADER – Lower Extremity Arterial Disease Event Reduction [trial]
LIPID – Long term Intervention with Pravastatin in Ischaemic Disease [trial]
LIPS – Lescol Intervention Prevention Study
LPL – lipoprotein lipase
LRC – Lipid Research Council
LRC-CPPT – Lipid Research Clinics – Coronary Primary Prevention Trial
MRFIT – Multiple Risk Factor Intervention Trial
MVE – major vascular event
NAFLD – non-alcoholic fatty liver disease
NCEP – National Cholesterol Education Program
NCEP ATP III – NCEP Adult Treatment Panel III
NEFA – non-esterified ('free') fatty acids
NNT – number needed to treat
PAD – peripheral arterial disease
POSCH – Program on the Surgical Control of the Hyperlipidemias
POST CABG – Post Coronary Artery Bypass Graft [trial]
PPAR-α – peroxisome proliferator-activated receptor alpha
PROGRESS – Perindopril Protection Against Recurrent Stroke Study

PROSPER – PROspective Study of Pravastatin in the Elderly at Risk [trial]
PROVE-IT – Pravastatin or Atorvastatin Evaluation and Infection Therapy [trial]
RCT – randomised controlled trial
ROS – reactive oxygen species
SEARCH – Study of Effectiveness of Additional Reductions of Cholesterol and Homocysteine [trial]
SHARP – Study of Heart and Renal Protection
SPARCL – Stroke Prevention by Aggressive Reduction in Cholesterol Levels [study]
SPPARM – selective peroxisome proliferator-activated receptor modulator

STARS – St Thomas' Atherosclerosis Regression Study
TexCAPS – Texas Coronary Atherosclerosis Prevention Study
TIA – transient ischaemic attack
TNT – Treating to New Targets [trial]
VA-HIT – Veterans Affairs High-Density Lipoprotein Cholesterol Intervention Trial
VLDL – very low density lipoprotein
WHO – World Health Organization
WOSCOPS – West of Scotland Coronary Prevention Study

LIST OF PATIENT QUESTIONS

CHAPTER 1

What are lipids?   14
Why is cholesterol important?   14
Where does cholesterol come from?   14
How much cholesterol do we need?   14
What is 'good' cholesterol?   15
What is 'bad' cholesterol?   15

CHAPTER 2

What is atherosclerosis?   33
What can happen to an atherosclerotic plaque?   33
What is cardiovascular disease?   34
How much do the major risk factors contribute to cardiovascular
disease?   35

CHAPTER 3

What is 'the lipid profile'?   44
How would I know if my lipid profile was abnormal?   45
What levels are desirable?   45

CHAPTER 4

At what age is cardiovascular disease considered premature? 61
How are the risks of passing on genetic hyperlipidaemia defined? 61
At what age should children be screened for genetic
hyperlipidaemia where there is a known family history?   63
Does identifying a genetic hyperlipidaemia make any difference? 64

CHAPTER 5

How can I get my cardiovascular risk assessed?   75
What is 'primary prevention'?   75
What is 'secondary prevention'?   76
What factors determine the level at which intervention is offered? 76

CHAPTER 6

How do I know if I am overweight?   94
How do I lose weight?   94
Is the 'Atkins' diet effective?   95
What are the most important dietary measures to prevent
cardiovascular disease?   95
How do I stick to a cardioprotective diet?   96
What is the safe limit for alcohol and which type should I drink? 96

What other measures should I take to prevent cardiovascular
disease?   97

CHAPTER 7
What alternative therapies are available for raised cholesterol and
blood fats?   124
Do drugs cure the problem?   124
At what time of day should lipid-lowering medication be taken?   125
Do lipid-lowering drugs cause impotence?   125
How do I know if lipid-lowering drugs are being effective?   125
What other drugs are advised in patients at high cardiovascular risk?   126

CHAPTER 8
Do clinical trials reflect the real world?   136
Would every adult benefit from a statin?   137

CHAPTER 9
Who should take 'over-the-counter' statins?   153

CHAPTER 10
Can you be too old for lipid-lowering treatment?   165
Do statins prevent dementia?   165
Does treatment for blood pressure affect lipid levels?   166
Do statins prevent osteoporosis?   166

CHAPTER 11
How can we afford lipid-lowering therapy?   170

INDEX

Note: Numbers in **bold** refer to
  boxes/figures/tables

A

Abdominal adiposity *see* Central adiposity;
    Waist circumference
Abetalipoproteinaemia, **49**
Absolute risk, 66
    compared with relative risk, 66
Acanthosis nigricans, 58, **59**
Acetyl CoA, metabolism, **8**
Achilles tendon xanthomata, in familial
    hypercholesterolaemia, 54, **54**
Acronyms (listed), 197–198
Adipose tissue
    atrophy, 59
    energy stored in, 2, 4
AFCAPS/TexCAPS (Air Force Coronary
    Atherosclerosis Prevention
    Study/Texas University Coronary
    Atherosclerosis Prevention Study),
    73, 132, **145**, **146**, **158**, **168**
African migrant populations, cardiovascular
    risks, 74
Alanine aminotransferase (ALT), levels
    during statin therapy, 107, 108
Alcohol consumption
    calculations, 96–97
    excess, effects, 92
    moderate, beneficial effects, 92, 93, 96
    type of alcohol, 97
Alpha-blockers, lipid levels affected by, 160,
    166
Alpha-linolenic acid, 87
Alternative treatments, 123–124
American Coronary Drug Project, 119
American Heart Association, dietary
    guidelines, 85, **86**
Angina (pectoris), 21, 33, 34
    Angiotensin converting enzyme (ACE)
        inhibitors, 127, 160, 166
    Angiotensin receptor blockers, 127, 160,
        166
Anglo-Scandinavian Cardiac Outcomes Trial
    (ASCOT), 45, 132, **145**, **146**, 160,
    166
Antihypertensive and Lipid Lowering
    treatment to prevent Heart Attack
    Trial (ALLHAT), **145**, 160, 166
Antihypertensive therapy, 126–127

lipid levels affected by, 160
Antioxidants, 93
    effect on heart disease, 93–94, 133
Antiretroviral agents
    interaction with statins, 106, 109, 163
    lipid levels affected by, **50**, 51–52, 163
Apolipoprotein-related Mortality Risk
    (AMORIS) study, 39
Apolipoproteins, 5, 6–8
    apo-A, 5, 6, **7**
    apo-B, 5, 6–8, **7**, 39
    apo-B48, 7, 9
    apo-B100, 7
    apo-C, 5, 8
    apo-CII, 8, 10
        deficiency, 60, 123
    apo-E, 5, 8
    measurement of, 39
    as risk indicators, 180
    role in body, 6–8
Arterial remodelling, 19, 21
Asian populations, cardiovascular risks, 30,
    74, 135
Aspirin, 126, 149
Assessment of LEscol in Renal
    Transplantation (ALERT) study, 109,
    132
Association of British Clinical Diabetologists
    (ABCD), contact information, 181
Atherogenesis, 18–20, **20**
    factors affecting, 11, 18
Atherogenic lipoprotein phenotype, 13
Atherogenic lipoprotein profile (ALP), 12, 13
Atherosclerosis, 33
    disorders resulting from, 33
    effect of HDL-cholesterol levels, 11–12
    effect of LDL-cholesterol levels, 11
    effect of triglycerides, 12–13
    risk factors, 12–13, 18
Atherosclerotic disease
    frequency of occurrence, 21
        population variations, **22**
    link with cholesterol levels, 21–22, **23**, **24**
Atherosclerotic plaque, formation, 18–19
Atkins diet, 95
Atorvastatin
    clinical trials/studies, 26, 28, 114,
        132–133, 134, 135, 161, 178
    combination with ezetimibe, 147
    dosage, 114
    efficacy, 111
    metabolism of, 106, 109, **110**, 113

Atorvastatin, *cont'd*
  side effects, **112**
  trials, 28
Audit systems, best practice implementation, 141
A-to-Z study, **146**, 178

B

'Bad' cholesterol, 11, 15–16
  see also LDL-cholesterol
Behaviour modification techniques, 94–95
Best practice
  guidelines, 141, **142**
  implementation of, 139–153
    obstacles to, 140–141
    underachievement, 140
    ways to achieve, 141
  pros and cons of targets, 142, 144
  target lipid levels, 141–142, **143**
    attainability, 147–148
    frequency of monitoring, 148
    strategies to achieve, 148
    total cholesterol vs LDL-cholesterol, 147
Beta-blockers
  lipid levels affected by, 50, **50**, 160, 166
  as protection against cardiovascular disease, 126
Bezafibrate, 116, 122, 161
Bile acid sequestrants, 102, 109, 120
  children treated with, 64
  in combination therapy, 121, 122
  interaction with other drugs, 125
  mode of action, 120
  side effects, 120
  timing of medication, 125
  see also Colestipol; Colestyramine
Bile acids/salts
  absorption of, 9
  chemical structure, **3**
  metabolism of, **9**
Blood pressure
  raised
    as risk factor, 12, 18, 21, 35
    treatment of, 159–160, 165–166
  (systolic) in risk assessment systems, **68–70, 71**
Blood Pressure Association, contact information, 181
Body mass index (BMI), 80–81
  threshold limits
    (normal/overweight/obese), 51, **80**, 94
British Cardiac Patients Association (BCPA), contact information, 181
British Cardiac Society (BCS), contact information, 181–182

British Diabetic Association *see* Diabetes UK
British Heart Foundation (BHF), contact information, 182
British Hyperlipidaemia Association *see* HEART UK
British Hypertension Society (BHS)
  contact information, 182
  guidelines, **142**, 160
British Regional Heart Study, 39, 67

C

C-reactive protein (CRP) levels
  effect of diet, 92
  effect of statins, 111, 178
Caerphilly study, 119
Calcification of arteries, measurement of, 73, 126
Calcium antagonists, 160, 166
Calorie-controlled diet, 94
Cancer deaths, effect of diet and lifestyle changes, 79–80
Cancer due to low cholesterol, 'risk' refuted, 27
Cannabinoid receptor blockers, 174, 177
Cardioprotective diet, 85
  adherence advice, 96
  LDL-cholesterol levels affected by, 26, 28, 130
Cardiovascular disease (CVD), 34
  effect of antioxidants, 93–94, 133
  effect of diet, 30, 85–88, 95–96
  effect of statins, 23, 133–134
  genetic factors, 31–32
    assessing genetic contribution, 31
    screening family members, 32
    specific single gene disorders, 31–32
  high-risk patients, **38**
  premature, 61
  protection measures, 126–127
  risk calculation, in Joint British Societies' guideline charts, 23, 61
  risk factors, 35, **71**
  variations between ethnic groups, 30–31
  variations between populations, factors affecting, 30
  see also Coronary heart disease; Stroke
Cardiovascular risk assessment
  accuracy, 67, 71–72
    ways of improving, 72–73
  global, 66
  individual, 66–67, **68–70**, 103
  risk factors included, **71**, 75
Cascade (genetic) screening, in UK, 32, 56
Central adiposity
  as risk factor, 13, 81
  see also Waist circumference

Cerebral thrombosis, 33
see also Stroke
Cerivastatin
interaction with gemfibrozil (fibrate), 106, 113
metabolism of, 106, 109, **110**, 113
side effects, 106, **112**, 113
withdrawal from use, 106, 113
Children
age at screening should be done, 63–64
drug therapy for, 64, 105, 156
lipid levels, 11, 24, 25, 28, 43, 135
Chinese populations, cholesterol levels, 11, 19, **24**, **26**
Cholesterol
absorption mechanism, 9–10
amount required by body, 15
chemical structure, 2, **3**, **88**
high levels
percentage population having, 27
as risk factor, 18, 21, 35
levels
CHD death rates affected by, 22, **23**, **24**, **25**
Chinese and Japanese populations, 11, 19, **24**, **26**, 29–30
'desirable' target, 45, 114, 135
effect of dietary fat intake, 82–83
effect of fasting, 39, 44
effect of statins, 103, 114
environmental factors affecting, 29
genetic/inherited variations, 29
in infants, 11, 24, 25, 28
in menopausal women on HRT, 159
methodological variations, 28–29
not affected by fasting, 39, 44
random variations, 28
ratio to HDL-cholesterol level, in JBS risk prediction charts, **69–70**
reasons for variation between individuals, 28–29
stroke risk affected by, 22–23
target, 27, 45, 114, 135, 142, **143**, 146–147
variations between populations, **23**, 29–30
low levels, risks refuted, 27–28, 130
measurement of *see* Lipid measurement
metabolism within cells, 10–11, 101, **102**
'normal' (typical) levels, 24–26
health-based definition, 25–26
in hunter–gatherer societies, 26, **26**
UK data, 25, **26**
in various populations, **26**
as precursor for other molecules, 2, **9**, 14
role in body, 2
sources, 8, 15
synthesis of, 8, **8**, **9**, **10**, 101

see also HDL-cholesterol; LDL-cholesterol
Cholesterol absorption inhibitors, 102, 117
see also Ezetimibe
Cholesterol ester transfer protein (CETP), 12
inhibitors, 124, 174, 175–176
Cholesterol lowering diet, 83, **84**
effect of medication affected by, 84
effectiveness, 83–84
Cholesterol and Recurrent Events (CARE) trial, 131, **145**, **146**, **158**, 163, 164, **168**
Chylomicrons, 4, 6, 9
Ciclosporin
interactions with statins, 106, 109, 163
lipid levels affected by, **50**, 51
Ciprofibrate, 116
Cis fatty acids, **3**
Classification of lipid disorders, 41, **42**
Clinical guidelines
future developments, 179–180
target lipid levels listed, 45, 114, 135, 142, **143**, 146–147
websites on, **142**, 184
see also European guidelines; Joint British Societies' guidelines; National Cholesterol Education Program (NCEP) guidelines
Clinical Resource Efficiency Support Team (CREST)
guidelines, **142**, 184
target lipid levels, **143**
Clinical trials, 129–137
early trials, 130
factors affecting, 136
fibrates, 134, 135, 161, **164**
limitations, 136
ongoing, 134–135, 178–179
issues to be addressed, 178–179
statins, 26, 28, 109, 114, 130–136, **145**, **146**, 161, 163, 164
Clopidogrel, as protection against cardiovascular disease, 126
Colestipol, 64, 120
Colestyramine, 64, 120
clinical trials, 28, 130
Collaborative Atorvastatin Diabetes Study (CARDS), 45, 133, **146**, 161
Combination therapy, 121–123
fibrates and ezetimibe, 118
fibrates and fish oil, 122, 123
fibrates and nicotinic acid, 122
preferred drug combinations, 122–123
statins and ezetimibe, 102, 115, 147, 148
statins and fibrates, 32, 106, 113, 116, 122, 148
statins and fish oil, 148
statins and nicotinic acid, 122, 148
statins and resins, 120, 122
when to be used, 121–122, 148

Combined hyperlipidaemia, **42**
Complex carbohydrates, in cholesterol-lowering diet, **84**, 91
Compliance considerations
  in clinical trials, 136
  in drug therapy, 115, 149
    factors affecting, 149
    tactics to enhance, 150, **150**
Computed tomography, 73
Conazoles, interaction with statins, 106, 109
Consensus guidelines *see* Clinical guidelines
Contraceptive pill, lipid levels affected by, 157–158
Coronary artery narrowing, measurement of, 126
Coronary calcification, measurement of, 73, 126
Coronary heart disease (CHD)
  heart failure caused by, 164
  rates
    Chinese and Japanese populations, 19, **22**, **23**
    effect of blood pressure, **25**
    effect of cholesterol levels, 22, **23**, **24**, **25**, 133, 134, **145**, **146**
    effect of diet, 85–88, 119
    effect of smoking, **25**
    effect of soy protein, 91
    effect of various drugs, 103, 119, 120
    in various countries, **22**, **23**
Coronary thrombosis, 33, 34
Cost considerations
  statin therapy, 105, 151, 170, 171
  see also Economic aspects
Cost-effectiveness
  primary prevention, 169–170
  secondary prevention, 169
Creatinine (phospho)kinase (CPK, CK), levels during statin therapy, 106, 108
Cytochrome P450 system, drugs metabolised through, 105–106, 109–110, **110**, 116

D

Dementia, effect of statins, 165
Diabetes mellitus
  cardiovascular disease and, 133, 134, 161
  as risk factor, 12, 18, 35
  treatment of, 121, 127
Diabetes UK, contact information, 182–183
Diabetic patients
  clinical trials/studies involving, 45, 133, 134, 135, **146**, 161, 179
  lipid lowering therapy for, 161–162
Diet
  cardiovascular disease rates affected by, 30, 85–88, 95–96

cholesterol levels affected by, 27, 82–84, 91–92
  see also Atkins diet; Cardioprotective diet; Cholesterol-lowering diet; Japanese diet; Mediterranean diet; 'Portfolio' diet
Diet and Reinfarction Trial (DART), 87
Dietary cholesterol intake, 15, 83
Dietary fats/triglycerides, 2
  digestion, 9
Dietary recommendations, **85**, **86**, 95–96
Disease states
  cholesterol levels affected by, 29
  hyperlipidaemias caused by, **48**, **49**, 50, **50**, 51
Diuretics, lipid levels affected by, 50, **50**, 52, 160, 166
Docosahexaenoic acid (DHA), 87
Drug interactions
  bile acid sequestrants, 125
  fibrates, 106, 116
  statins, 32, 106, 109–110, 113, 116, 117, 163
Drug therapies
  for cardiovascular high risk patients, 126–127
  clinical trial evidence, 129–137
  hyperlipidaemia(s) caused by, 50–51, **50**, 51–52
  for lipid disorders, 99–127
    alternative treatments, 123–124
    and cholesterol-lowering diet, 84, 124
    clinical trial evidence, 129–137
    combination therapy, 121–123
    compliance considerations, 115
    fibrates, 115–117
    monitoring of effectiveness, 126
    other pharmacological treatments, 117–121
    statins, 101–115
  timing of medication, 125
  see also Treatment
Durrington's classification of dyslipidaemias, 41, **42**
Dysbetalipoproteinaemia, familial, 29, 32
Dyslipidaemias, 18, 41
  primary, classification, 41, **42**, **48–49**
  see also Hypercholesterolaemia; Hypertriglyceridaemia

E

Economic aspects, 167–171
  see also Cost considerations
Egg consumption, 15, 83
Eicosapentanoic acid (EPA), 87
Elaidic acid, chemical structure, **3**
Electrophoresis, lipoproteins classified by, 6

Endothelial damage
  causes, 35
  events resulting from, 19, 20, 33, 34
Enterocyte
  cholesterol absorbed via, 9–10
  effect of ezetimibe, 10, 117
Environmental factors affecting cholesterol
    levels, 29, 30
Eruptive (skin) xanthomata, 58, **59**
Erythromycin, interaction with statins, 106,
    109
Ethnicity
  cardiovascular disease rates, 30–31
    quantification in risk assessment
      systems, 74
EUROASPIRE 2, 140
European guidelines, **142**
  basis, 67
  risk assessment charts, **70**
  risk factors included, **71**
  target lipid levels, **143**, 146, 180
  treatment threshold, 74
European Society of Cardiology (ESC)
    guidelines, **142**, 185
  target lipid levels, **143**
Exercise, effect on cholesterol levels, 27
Exercise-induced myocardial ischaemia, 21
Ezetimibe, 102, 117–118
  children treated with, 64
  combination with other drugs, 102, 118,
    121, 122, 147, 148
  dosage, 117
  mode of action, 10, 117
  side effects, 118

F

Familial combined hyperlipidaemia, **42**, **49**,
    56, 156
  referral to specialist clinic, 151
Familial defective apolipoprotein-B (FDB),
    42, **48**, 52, 56
Familial dysbetalipoproteinaemia, 29, 32, **42**,
    49, 56–58
  referral to specialist clinic, 151
  treatment of, 32, 58, 64, 116
  see also Hyperlipidaema, type III; Remnant
    particle disease
Familial hypercholesterolaemia (FH), 18, 29,
    31–32, **48**, 49, 52–53, 121
  diagnosis of children, 63, 156
  diagnostic features, 53–56, **53**
  further diagnosis of cases, 55–56
  gene replacement therapy for, 174, 177
  genetic risks, 52–53, 62
  prevalence, **42**, 52, 53, 62, 63
  referral to specialist clinic, 151
  screening for, 32, 55–56, 63, 64

treatment of children, 63–64, 156
treatment by diet and lifestyle changes,
    80
treatment by drugs, 103, 120, 121
treatment by LDL-apheresis, 123
women on contraceptive pill, 157–158
Familial hypertriglyceridaemia, **42**, 49
Familial phytosterolaemia, 89–90
Family history of cardiovascular disease, 31,
    73, 75
  and genetic considerations, 31–32
Family screening, 31–32, 52, 56, 63, 64
Fasting, triglyceride levels affected by, 39,
    44
Fasting lipid profile, 44, 126
Fat
  dietary intake, 82–83
  energy density, 82
Fatty acids, 4, 86
  chemical structure, **3**, **5**, 86
  monounsaturated fatty acids, 4, 82
  non-esterified (free) fatty acids, 2, 5,
    119
  polyunsaturated fatty acids, 4, 82, 86–87
Fatty streak
  foam cells, 11, 19, 20
  ground substance, 19
Fenofibrate, 32, 58, 116, 117
  clinical trials/studies, 134, 135, 161, 179
  in combination with statins, 106, 117, 121,
    122
Fenofibrate Intervention and Event
    Lowering in Diabetes (FIELD) study,
    134, 135, 161, 179
Fibrates, 13, 109, 115–117
  clinical trials/studies, 134, 135, 161, **164**,
    179
    heart failure development in, **164**
  combination with other drugs, 118, 122,
    123, 124
  combination with statins, 32, 106, 113,
    116, 121, 122, 147
  contraindications, 163
  diabetic dyslipidaemia treated with, 161
  efficacy, 116–117
  hypertriglyceridaemia treated with, 60,
    116, 122
  indications for, 115–116
  interactions with other drugs, 106, 116
  mode of action, 115
  remnant hyperlipidaemia treated with, 32,
    58, 64, 116
  see also Familial dysbetaliporoteinaemia;
    Hyperlipidaemia, type III, Remnant
    particle disease
  side effects, 116, 117
  timing of medication, 125
  see also Bezafibrate; Ciprofibrate;
    Fenofibrate; Gemfibrozil

Fish, in diet, 87, 119
Fish oil capsules, 88, 119, 148
　combination with other drugs, 122, 123,
　　148
　hypertriglyceridaemia treated with, 60,
　　119, 122, 124
Fluvastatin
　clinical trials/studies, 109, 132, 163
　dosage, 114
　efficacy, 111
　metabolism of, 106, 109, **110**, 113
　side effects, **112**
Folic acid
　in multi-medication, 149
　supplementation study, 18
Food labelling, 85, **87**
Framingham study, 22, **24**, 66, 71
　risk assessment system, 66, 67
　　accuracy, 67
　　adjustment factor for non-Caucasian
　　　populations, 74
　　shortcomings, 71–72
Friedewald formula, 40
Future developments, 173–180

G

Gastrointestinal disease, effect of diet and
　lifestyle changes, 80
Gemfibrozil
　avoidance in combination with statins, 32,
　　106, 113, 116
　clinical trials, 28, 130
　side effects, 116, 117
Gender differences
　cardiovascular disease rates, 30, 35
　lipid levels, 43, **44**
Gene replacement therapy, 123, 124, 174,
　177–178
General Medical Services (GMS) contract,
　103, 141, 148
　inappropriateness of targets, 144
Genetic factors, cholesterol levels affected by,
　29, 31–32
Genetic hyperlipidaemia
　advantages of identifying, 64
　age at which children should be screened,
　　63–64
　drug therapy for children, 156
　risks, 61–63
　see also Familial hypercholesterolaemia;
　　Hyperlipidaemia, type III, Remnant
　　particle disease
Genetic screening, in UK, 32, 56
GISSI-Prevenzione trial, 119
Glitazones, 121, 176
Global cardiovascular disease assessment,
　66

Global risk factor modification, 148–149
　for hypertensive patients, 160
Glossary, 197–198
Glucose intolerance, as risk factor, 12, 18
Glycerol, 2, 10
'Good' cholesterol, 11–12, 15
　see also HDL-cholesterol
Gout, in insulin resistance/metabolic
　syndrome, 13, 31
Grapefruit juice, drug metabolism affected
　by, 109
GREek Atorvastatin and Coronary heart
　disease Evaluation (GREACE) study,
　146, 147, **164**
Guidelines see Clinical guidelines

H

Haemodialysis patients, lipid lowering
　therapy for, 162
HDL-cholesterol
　atherosclerosis affected by, 11–12
　elevation of, 174, 175–176
　levels
　　'desirable' level, 45, 147
　　effect of fibrates, 115, 117
　　effect of nicotinic acid, 120
　　effect of statins, 110–111
　　gender differences, 43, **44**
　　in menopausal women on HRT,
　　　159
　　not affected by fasting, 39, 44
　　variation with age, 43, **44**
　see also High density lipoproteins
'Heart attack', 33, 34
　treatment of, 34
　see also Coronary thrombosis; Myocardial
　　infarction
Heart failure patients, lipid lowering therapy
　for, 164–165
Heart Protection Study (HPS), 28, 38, 40,
　45, 133–134, 144, **145**, **146**, 163–164,
　179–180
　on cost–benefit considerations, 170–171
　diabetic patients in, 134, 161
　older people in, 156, 157, 165
　women in, 157
HEART UK, 55, 183
Helsinki Heart Study (HHS), 28, 116, 130
Hepatic disease, hyperlipidaemia caused by,
　50, 51
High density lipoproteins (HDLs), 11–12
　components, 5, 6, **7**
　role in body, 11, 12, 15
　synthesis, 11
　synthetic, 175
　see also HDL-cholesterol
High protein diet, 95

HIV patients, lipid lowering therapy for, 163
Homocysteine levels, elevated, 18
Hormone replacement therapy (HRT), lipid levels affected by, 159
3-Hydroxy-3-methylglutaryl-coenzyme-A (HMG-CoA) reductase, 8, **8**, **10**
  inhibition by statins, **8**, **10**, 101, 110
Hypercholesterolaemia
  combined with hypertriglyceridaemia, **42**
  familial, 18, 29, 31–32, **48**, 49, 53–56
    see also Familial hypercholesterolaemia
  as risk factor, 18, 21, 35
  treatment by diet, 82, 84, 89, 91, 92
  treatment by drugs, 110–111, 114, 115, 116, 117, 118, 120, 122
  see also Dyslipidaemia
Hyperlipidaemia(s)
  primary, 48, **48**, 49–50
  secondary, 48, **48**, 49, 50–51, **50**
  type I, 49
  type II, **42**, 49, 55
  type III, 29, 32, **42**, 49–50, **49**, 56–58
    referral to specialist clinic, 151
    treatment of, 32, 58, 64, 116
    see also Familial dysbetalipoproteinaemia; Remnant particle disease
  type IV, **42**, 50, 55
  type V, **42**, 49
  see also Dyslipidaemia(s)
Hypertension, as risk factor, 12, 18, 21, 35
Hypertensive patients, lipid lowering therapy for, 159–160, 165–166
Hypertriglyceridaemia, **42**, **48**, 49, 121
  combined with hypercholesterolaemia, **42**
  isolated, 58–60
  treatment of, 60, 115, 116, 119, 122
Hypertriglyceridaemic waist phenotype, 81
Hyperuricaemia
  in insulin resistance/metabolic syndrome, 13, 31
  as risk factor, 13
Hypoalphalipoproteinaemia, **42**
Hypobetalipoproteinaemia, **42**, **49**

I

Identifying patients for treatment, 65–76
Implementation of best practice, obstacles to, 140–141
Impotence, causes, 125–126
Incremental Decrease in Endpoints through Aggressive Lipid lowering (IDEAL) trial, 114, 134, 178
Indian subcontinent populations
  BMI thresholds, 51

insulin resistance syndrome, 31
Infants, cholesterol levels, 11, 24, 25, 28, 135
'Influenza like' (muscle) symptoms, in statin therapy, 106, 107, 108
Inherited factors affecting cholesterol levels, 29
Inherited hyperlipidaemia *see* Genetic hyperlipidaemia
Inherited risk factors, 18
Insulin resistance
  clinical signs, 58–59
  as risk factor, 21
Insulin resistance syndrome, 12–13
  research into, 178–179
  in South Asian populations, 30, 31
  see also Metabolic syndrome
Insulin sensitisers, 121, 176–177
  clinical trials, 179
INTERHEART case-control study, 39, 73
Intermediate density lipoproteins (IDLs), 10, 56
Intermittent claudication, 34, 162
Intervention, factors determining level at which offered, 76, 103
Isolated hypertriglyceridaemia, 58–60
  diagnostic features, 58–59
Isoprenoid units, **8**, **9**

J

Japanese diet, 85
Japanese populations
  CHD rates, **22**
    effect of lifestyle changes, 31, 135
  cholesterol levels, 11, 19, **26**, 29
    effect of lifestyle changes, 19, 29–30, 135
  waist circumference thresholds, 51
Joint British Societies (JBS)
  guidelines, **142**
    basis, 67
    and genetic contributions, 31, 73
    and premature cardiovascular disease, 61
    risk factors included, **71**
    target lipid levels, 114, 135, **143**, 146–147, 180
    treatment threshold, 74, 103, 104
    web page, 31, 135
  risk assessment charts, 23, **68–69**, 74, 103, 104
  see also British Cardiac Society; British Hyperlipidaemia Association; British Hypertension Society; Diabetes UK; HEART UK; Primary Care Cardiovascular Society; Stroke Association
Journals (listed), 186

L

LDL-apheresis (therapy), 123
LDL-cholesterol
  atherosclerosis and, 11
  levels
    cardiovascular risk affected by, 26, 28,
      130, 133, 134
    effect of diet, 82, 84, 92, 124
    effect of ezetimibe, 118, 124
    effect of fibrates, 117
    effect of plant sterols, 89, 124
    effect of resins, 120, 124
    effect of soy protein, 91
    effect of statins, 110–111, 114, 115, 116,
      124, **146**, 156
    gender differences, 43, **44**
    in infants, 11, 25, 28, 135
    measurement/calculation of, 40, 126, 144
    in menopausal women on HRT, 159
    population variation, 11
    target, 45, 114, 135, **143**, 145
    variation with age, 43, **44**
    in various clinical trials, **146**
  metabolism of, 11, 19
  see also Low density lipoproteins
Lecithin cholesterol acyl transferase (LCAT,
    enzyme), 11, 12
  deficiency, **49**
Lescol Intervention Prevention Study (LIPS),
    132, **146**
Life expectancy, 61
  in familial hypercholesterolaemia, 52, 53
Lifestyle changes
  cholesterol levels affected by, 27, 124
  in Japanese populations, 19, 29–30
  Prochaska and DiClemente's model, **79**
Lifestyle factors, cholesterol levels affected by,
    29
Lifestyle Heart Trial, 79
Linolenic acid, 87
Lipid disorders, 47–64
  classification, 41, **42**, **48–49**
  identifying individuals for treatment,
    65–76
  treatment by diet and lifestyle, 77–97
  treatment by drugs, 99–127
    clinical trial evidence, 129–137
Lipid measurement, 37–45, 126
  accuracy, 41, 43
  frequency of repeat testing, 43, 148
  individuals to be tested, 38
  lipid abnormalities seen, 40–41, 45
  location of testing, 38–39
  statin therapy and, 104
  tests to be done, 39
Lipid metabolism, overview, 1–16

Lipid profile, 39, 44–45
  abnormalities in, 40–41, 45
  desirable/target values, 45, **143**, 146–147
  effect of diet, 84, 87
  effect of physical activity, 82
  gender differences, 43, **44**
  variations with age, 43, **44**
Lipid Research Clinics – Coronary Primary
    Prevention Trial (LRC-CPPT), 28,
    120, 130, **146**
Lipid Research Council study, **145**
Lipid Treatment Assessment Project, 140
Lipidologist, specialist, 60–61, 150–151
Lipids, meaning of term, 14
Lipoprotein lipase (LPL, enzyme)
  action, 8, 10
  activation of, 8, 10
  inherited absence, 12, 60
Lipoprotein lipase deficiency, **42**, 49, 60
  gene replacement therapy for, 123, 124,
    174, 177–178
  treatment of, 60, 123
Lipoproteins, 5
  classification of, 6
  high density, 11–12
  lipoprotein(a) (Lp(a)), 13–14
  low density, 4, 6, 10
  metabolism, 10–11
  physical structure, **7**
  protein components, 6–8
  solubilisation in blood, 5
  types, 5
Liver disease, hyperlipidaemia caused by, **50**,
    51
Liver enzymes, disturbance due to statin
    therapy, 106–107, 109, 114
Long-term Intervention with Pravastatin in
    Ischaemic Disease (LIPID) trial, 131,
    145, **146**, **158**, 163, **168**
Lovastatin
  efficacy, 111
  metabolism of, 106, 109, **110**, 113
  side effects, **112**, 158
Low carbohydrate diet, 95
Low density lipoproteins (LDLs), 4, 6,
    10
  effect of excess levels, 11, 16
  role in body, 11, 15–16, 101
  triglyceride-enriched, 13, 115
  see also LDL-cholesterol
Low fat diets, 60, 84, **84**, 123
Low levels of cholesterol, risks refuted,
    27–28, 130
Low lipid/lipoprotein levels, dyslipidaemias
    with, **49**
Lower Extremity Arterial Disease Event
    Reduction (LEADER) trial, 162
Lyon Diet Heart Study, 85, 87

M

Mediterranean diet, 85, **85**
Menopause, lipid levels in, 159
Metabolic syndrome, 51, 81
    future treatments, 176
    NCEP definition, **13**, 51, 176
    research into, 178–179
    see also Insulin resistance syndrome
Metformin, 121, 178–179
Methodological variations in cholesterol
        levels, 28–29
Mixed hyperlipidaemia, **49**, 121
    factors affecting, 32, **49**
    referral to specialist clinic, 151
    in South Asian populations, 30, 31
    treatment of, 115, 116, 119, 122, 176
Monogenic hypercholesterolaemia, **42**
Monounsaturated fatty acids, 4, 82
    in Mediterranean diet, **85**
Multidisciplinary approach to best practice,
        141
Multi-medication approach, 149
Multiple Risk Factor Intervention Trial
        (MRFIT), 22, **25**, 27, 130
Myalgia
    management of, 108
    as side effect of statin therapy, **112**
Myocardial infarction, 21
Myocardial ischaemia, exercise-induced, 21
Myopathy
    causes, 107
    as side effect of statin therapy, 106, **112**
Myositis, as side effect of drug therapy, 105,
        112, 113, 116, 122

N

n-3 fatty acids, 86–87
    benefits, 87–88
National Assembly for Wales
    contact information, 184
    guidelines, **142**
    target lipid levels, **143**
National Cholesterol Education Program
        (NCEP)
    Adult Treatment Panel III (ATP-III)
        guidelines, 45, **71**, 74, 116, 135, 142
        non-HDL cholesterol target, 147
        target lipid levels, 45, 135, 142, **143**, 147
        web page, **142**
    on compliance improvement, 150, **150**
    on metabolic syndrome, **13**, 51, 136, 176
    recommendations on screening, 38, **40**
    risk assessment system
        basis, 67
        risk factors included, **71**
        treatment threshold, 74
National Obesity Forum (NOF), contact
        information, 183
National Service Framework (NSF)
    for Coronary Heart Disease, 103, **142**,
        184
        target lipid levels, **143**
    for Diabetes, 103, 184
Nicotinic acid, 109, 119
    in combination therapy, 122, 148
    hypertriglyceridaemia treated with, 60,
        119, 122
    side effects, 119–120
    timing of medication, 125
Non-alcoholic fatty liver diseases (NAFLD),
        107, 114
Non-Caucasian populations, adjustment
        factor in risk assessment systems, 74
Non-esterified/free fatty acids (NEFA), 2, 5
    levels, reduction of, 119
Non-HDL cholesterol, 147
    target levels, 146, 147
'Number needed to treat' (NNT), 168
    figures from major statin trials, **168**

O

Obesity
    factors affecting, 81, 83
    in insulin resistance/metabolic syndrome,
        31
    as risk factor, 13
    see also Body mass index (BMI); Central
        adiposity
Odds ratio (OR), 73
Oestrogens, lipid levels affected by, **50**, 51,
        158
Older people
    age at which lipid-lowering therapy
        started, 165
    clinical trials involving, **145**, **146**, 156, 157,
        165
    dementia risks, 165
    effectiveness of statins, 156–157, 165
Oleic acid, chemical structure, **3**
Omacor fish oil supplement, 119
Omega-3 fatty acids, 86–87
    benefits, 87–88
Omega-3 fish oil capsules, 119
    combination with other drugs, 122, 123
Ongoing clinical trials, 134–135, 178–179
    issues to be addressed, 178–179
Osteoporosis, effect of statins, 166
'Over the counter' (OTC) statins, 74,
        103–104, 125, 137, 151–153
    cholesterol measurement and, 104, 153

'Over the counter', *cont'd*
  concerns about, 152, **152**
  cost considerations, 151, 171
  individuals who could benefit, 103–104,
    125, 137, 151, 153

P

Palmar crease xanthomata, in type III
    hyperlipidaemia, 57, **57**
Pancreatitis, hypertriglyceridaemia and, 58,
    116, 123
Perindopril Protection Against Recurrent
    Stroke Study (PROGRESS), 149
Peripheral arterial disease (PAD) patients,
    lipid lowering therapy for, 162
Peroxisome proliferator-activated receptors
    (PPARs), 115, 176–177
  see also Selective PPAR modulators
Pharmacist-controlled supply of statins, 74,
    103–104, 125, 137, 151–153
Pharmacy testing (of cholesterol levels), 29,
    39
Phospholipids, 4
Physical activity
  advice on, 82, 97
  lipid profile affected by, 82
Phytosterols (plant sterols), 88–89
Plant sterols and stanols, 88–89, 109
  chemical structures, **88**
  LDL-cholesterol levels affected by, 89, 124
  mechanism of action, 89
  safety, 89–90
  spreads/margarines containing, 89, 124
  who should use, 90
Plaque, atherosclerotic
  formation, 18–19
  rupture, 20, **20**
    consequences, 21
  vulnerable plaque, 19–20
Plasminogen, and lipoprotein(a), 14
'Pleiotropic' effects of statins, 101, 111
Polygenic hypercholesterolaemia, **42**, **48**, 52
  genetic considerations, 52, 63
'Polypill', 149
Polyunsaturated fatty acids, 4, 82, 86–87
Population attributable risk (PAR), 73
  listed for various risk factors, **72**
'Portfolio' diet, 91–92
Pravastatin
  clinical trials, 26, 28, 114, 131, 135, **145**,
    146, 156, 157, **158**, 163, 165, **168**,
    178
  dosage, 114
  efficacy, 111
    for older people, 157
  metabolism of, 106, 109, **110**, 113
  side effects, **112**

Pravastatin or Atorvastatin Evaluation and
    Infection Therapy (PROVE-IT) trial,
    26, 28, 114, 135, **146**, 178
Pregnancy, lipid-lowering drugs and, 64, 105,
    158–159
Premature cardiovascular disease, 61
  risk assessment adjustment for, 73
Premature corneal arcus, 55, 56, 57
Primary cardiovascular disease prevention,
    38–39
Primary Care Cardiovascular Society
    (PCCS), contact information, 183
Primary hyperlipidaemias, 48, **48–49**, 49–50
Primary prevention, 74, 75, 103
  cost-effectiveness, 169–170
  lipid measurement in, 104
  percentage of population in UK, 170
  studies/trials, 132–133
Progestins, lipid levels affected by, 158
Program on the Surgical Control of the
    Hyperlipidaemias (POSCH), **145**
PROspective Study of Pravastatin in the
    Elderly at Risk (PROSPER) trial,
    145, **146**, 156, 157, 165
Protease inhibitors
  interaction with statins, 106, 109, 163
  lipid levels affected by, **50**, 52, 163

Q

Quebec Heart Study, 39

R

Radical therapy, 123–124
Random variations in cholesterol levels, 28
Reactive oxygen species (ROS), 93
Relative risk, compared with absolute risk, 66
Remnant(s), 10, 56
Remnant hyperlipidaemia/lipidaemia *see*
    Remnant particle disease
Remnant particle disease (remnant lipaemia),
    29, 32, **42**, **49**, 56–58
  diagnostic features, 57, 62
  genetic background, 57–58, 62–63
  prevalence, **42**, 62
  treatment of, 32, 58, 64, 116
  see also Familial dysbetalipoproteinaemia,
    Hyperlipidaemia, type III
Renal disease
  chronic, lipid lowering therapy used,
    162–163
  lipid levels affected by, **50**, 51, 162–163
Resins, 120
  children treated with, 64, 156
  in combination therapy, 121, 122, 148
  see also Bile acid sequestrants

Retinoic acid, hyperlipidaemia caused by, **50**, 51
Retroviral agents/therapy *see* Antiretroviral agents
Rhabdomyolysis, as side effect of statin therapy, 105, **112**, 113
Risk
  absolute, 66
    assessment for individual, 66–67
    compared with relative risk, 66
Risk assessment
  accuracy, 67, 71–72
    ways of improving, 72–73
  factors affecting, 67
  global, 66
  individual, 66–67, **68–70**, 103, 125, 137
    risk factors included, **71**, 75
Risk factors, 12–13, 18, 21–22, 35, 80, 81
  effect of genetic contribution, 31
  effect of lipoprotein(a) levels, 14
  environmentally influenced, 18
  inherited, 18
  in various risk assessment systems, **71**
Rosuvastatin
  efficacy, 111, 147
  metabolism of, 106, 109–110, **110**
  side effects, 107
Royal College of Physicians (RCP), contact information, 184

S

Safety monitoring, of statin therapy, 108
St Thomas' Atherosclerosis Regression Study (STARS), 120, 130
Scandinavian Simvastatin Survival Study (4S), 114, 130–131, **145**, **146**, **158**, 163, **164**, **168**, 169
Scottish Health Survey data, 73–74
Scottish Intercollegiate Guidelines Network (SIGN), **142**, 184
  target lipid levels, **143**
Screening, genetic, 32
SEARCH study, 18, 114
Seasonal variations in cholesterol levels, 29
Secondary hyperlipidaemia(s), 48, **48**, **49**
  conditions causing, 50–51, **50**
  drugs causing, **50**, 51–52
Secondary prevention, 76, 103, 179
  cost-effectiveness, 169
  percentage of population in UK, 170
  studies/trials, 131–132
Selective (o)estrogen receptor modulators (SERMs), 159
Selective PPAR modulators (SPPARMs), 174, 177
Seven Countries Study, 22, **23**
Side effects

bile acid sequestrants, 120
  ezetimibe, 118
  fibrates, 106, 116
  nicotinic acid, 119–120
  statins, 106–107
'Silent' lesions, 19
Simvastatin, 104
  clinical trials/studies, 114, 130–131, 133, 134, **145**, **146**, **158**, 163, **164**, **168**, 169
  combination with ezetimibe, 122
  dosage, 114
  efficacy, 111
  metabolism of, 106, 109, **110**, 113
  'over the counter' availability, 104, 137, 151
  side effects, **112**, 158
Single gene disorders, 31–32
  gene replacement therapy for, 123, 124, 174, 177–178
  see also Familial dysbetalipoproteinaemia; Familial hypercholesterolaemia
Sitostanol, **88**
β-Sitosterol, **88**
Smoking
  advice on, 97, 158
  gender differences, 30
  heart disease mortality affected by, **25**, 97
  as risk factor, 18, 21
South Asian populations, cardiovascular risks, 30, 74, 135
Soy isoflavones, 91
Soy protein, 91–92
  cholesterol-lowering properties, 91
Specialist secondary care centres, 60, 123
  patients who should be referred, 150–151
Statin–fibrate combination therapy, 32
  avoidance of cerivastatin–gemfibrozil, 32, 106, 116
Statins, 101–115
  alternative treatments, 109
  augmentation by dietary changes, 101–102
  children treated with, 64, 105, 156
  clinical trials/studies, 26, 28, 109, 114, 130–136, **145**, **146**, **158**, 161, 163, 164, **164**, **168**
    heart failure development in, **164**
    women, **158**
  combination with other drugs, 102, 115, 118, 120, 121, 122, 123, 147, 148
    gemfibrozil to be avoided, 32, 106, 113, 116, 117
  contraindications, 105–106
  cost considerations, 105, 151, 169–170, 171
  dementia affected by, 165
  diabetic dyslipidaemia treated with, 161
  dosage, 114
  efficacy of various statins, 110–111

Statins, *cont'd*
  factors limiting use, 105–106, 108–109
  future developments, 173–174
  indications for, 32, 58, 102–103
  individuals identified for treatment,
    102–104, 137
  interactions with other drugs, 32, 106,
    109–110, 113, 116, 117, 163
  LDL-cholesterol reduction using,
    110–111, 114, 115, 116, 124, **146**,
    156
  lipid measurement prior to initiation,
    104–105
  metabolism of, 105–106, 109–110, 113
  mode of action, **8**, **10**, 101–102
  osteoporosis affected by, 166
  'over the counter' availability, 74, 103–104,
    125, 137, 151–153
  'pleiotropic' effects, 101, 111
  poor response to treatment, 115
  pregnancy and, 64, 105, 158–159
  remnant lipaemia treated with, 32, 58
  see also Familial dysbetalipoproteinaemia,
    Hyperlipidaemia, type III
  safety monitoring for, 108
  side effects, 106–107, 111–113
    alternative statin switched to, 113
  stroke incidence reduced by, 23, 149,
    163–164
  time to be effective, 103, 105
  timing of medication, 125
  see also Atorvastatin; Cerivastatin;
    Fluvastatin; Lovastatin; Pravastatin;
    Rosuvastatin; Simvastatin
Stearic acid, chemical structure, **3**
Steroid nucleus, chemical structure, **3**
Sterols, chemical structures, **3**, **88**
Stroke, 21, 33, 34
  risk due to raised cholesterol levels, 22–23
  reduction of, 23, 149, 163–164
Stroke patients, lipid lowering therapy for,
  163–164
Study of Effectiveness of Additional
    Reductions of Cholesterol and
    Homocysteine (SEARCH) trial, 134,
    178
Systematic Coronary Risk Evaluation
    (SCORE) system, 67, 72

T

Tachyphylaxis, 115, 148
Tamoxifen, 159
Tangier disease, **49**
Target lipid levels
  attainability, 147–148
  frequency of checking, 148
  percentage reduction targets, **143**, 144
  pros and cons, 142, 144
  strategies to achieve, 148
  various recommendations, 45, 114, 135,
    142, **143**, 146–147
Tendon xanthomata, in familial
    hypercholesterolaemia, 53, 54, **54**
Thiazides (diuretics), lipid levels affected by,
  50, **50**, 52, 160, 166
Thiazolidinediones, 60, 121, 174, 176
  clinical trials, 179
Thrombosis, 21, 33, 34
Titration, 148
Tobacco use *see* Smoking
Torcetrapib (CETP inhibitor), 175, 176,
  179
Trans fatty acids, **3**, 82
Transaminases, increase due to statin therapy,
  107, 109, 114
Treating to New Targets (TNT) trial, 26, 28,
  114, 135, **146**, 178
Treatment
  by diet and lifestyle, 77–97
  by drugs, 99–127
    alternative treatments, 123–124
    clinical trial evidence, 129–137
    combination therapy, 121–123
    compliance considerations, 115
    fibrates, 115–117
    other pharmacological treatments,
      117–121
    statins, 101–115
  identifying individuals for, 65–76, 125,
    137
  threshold for initiation, 73–74
Triglyceride-enriched low density
    lipoproteins, 13, 115
Triglycerides, 2
  absorption mechanism, 9
  atherosclerosis affected by, 12–13
  chemical structure, **5**
  hydrolysis, 8, 10
  levels
    'desirable' threshold, 45
    effect of fasting, 39, 44
    effect of fibrates, 115, 116, 117, 124,
      163
    effect of fish oil, 119, 124, 163
    effect of nicotinic acid, 119, 124
    high levels, 27, **42**
    in menopausal women on HRT,
      159
    'normal' (typical) levels, 24, 27, **42**
  metabolism, 4
  role in body, 4
  sources, 2, 4
Tubular proteinuria, in statin therapy,
  107
Type I hyperlipidaemia, 49
Type II hyperlipidaemia, **42**, 49, 55

Type III hyperlipidaemia, 29, 32, **42**, 49–50,
    49, 56–58
    referral to specialist clinic, 151
    treatment of, 32, 58, 64, 116
    see also Familial dysbetalipoproteinaemia,
        Remnant particle disease
Type IV hyperlipidaemia, **42**, 50, 55
Type V hyperlipidaemia, **42**, 49

U

UK
    CHD mortality data, **22**
    CVD/lipid guidelines, 114, 135, **143**,
        146–147, 180
    genetic (cascade) screening, 32, 56, 64
    typical cholesterol levels, 24, **25**
Ultracentrifugation, lipoproteins classified by,
    6
Ultrasound techniques, 73, 126
Undertreatment, 140
Unsaturated fatty acids, 4
USA
    CHD mortality data, **22**, **23**, **25**
    NCEP guidelines, 45, **71**, 74, 116, 135,
        142, 180
        target lipid levels, 45, 135, 142, **143**, 147
    typical cholesterol levels, **26**

V

'Very high risk' patients, definition, 142
Very low density lipoproteins (VLDLs), 4, 6,
    10, 101
    suppression of hepatic secretion, 115
    see also VLDL-cholesterol
Very low fat diets, 60, 123
Veterans Affairs High-density lipoprotein
    cholesterol Intervention Trial
    (VA-HIT), 116, 161, **164**
Vitamin D, chemical structure, **3**
Vitamin supplements, effect on heart disease,
    93, 133
VLDL-cholesterol, 40, 147
Vulnerable plaque, 19–20

W

Waist circumference
    in Asian populations, 51, **81**
    in insulin resistance/metabolic syndrome,
        13, 31, 51, 81
    obesity-related complications and, **81**

Wanless Report, on cost of statin therapy,
    171
Warfarin
    interaction with statins, 110
    as protection against cardiovascular disease,
        126
Websites
    government sites, 184
    patient information, 181–184, 185–186
    research sites, 184–185
Weight, threshold limits
        (normal/overweight/obese), 51, **80**,
        94
Weight loss
    benefits, 81–82
    how to achieve, 94–95
Weight reduction drugs, 127, 177
Weight/height relationship, **80**, 94
    see also Body mass index
Welsh Assembly
    guidelines, **142**, 184
    target lipid levels, **143**
West of Scotland Coronary Prevention Study
        (WOSCOPS), 132, **145**, **146**, **168**,
        169
Women
    cardiovascular disease risk, 157
        effect of lipid-lowering therapy, 157,
            158
    menopausal, 159
    osteoporosis in, 166
Women's Health Initiative trial, 159
World Health Organization (WHO)
    lipid disorders classification, 41, **42**
    weight classification, 94

X

Xanthelasma(ta), 55, **55**, 56, 57
Xanthomata *see* Eruptive xanthomata; Palmar
        crease xanthomata; Tendon
        xanthomata